KU-452-811

CORE STRENGTH TRAINING

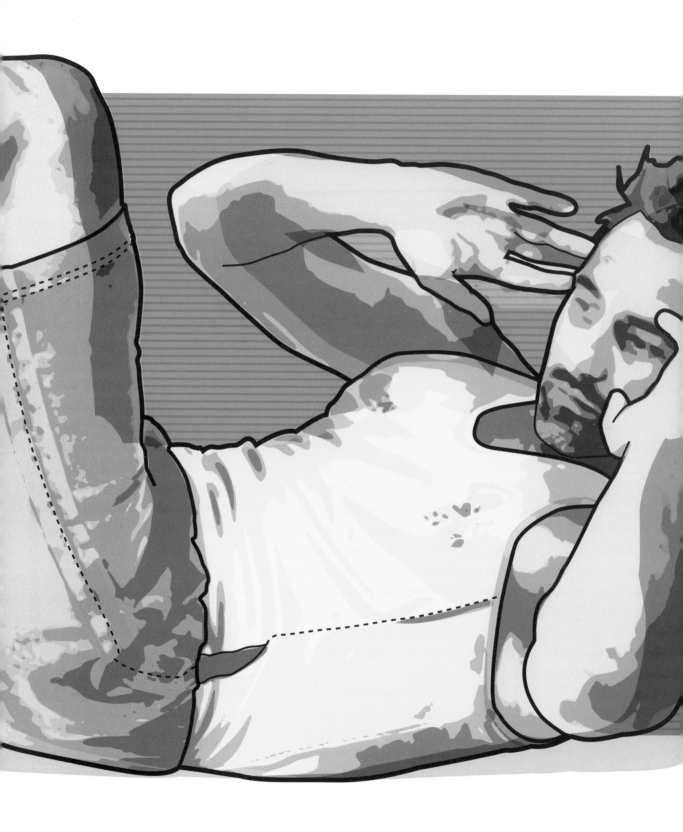

CORE
STRENGTH
TRAINING

The Complete Step-by-Step Guide to a Stronger Body and Better Posture for Men and Women

LONDON, NEW YORK, MUNICH,
MELBOURNE, DELHI

Senior Editor	Gareth Jones
Editorial team	Andy Szudek, Hugo Wilkinson, Kajal Mistry, Peter Preston, Chris Stone, Satu Fox
Project Art Editor	Katie Cavanagh
Design team	Keith Davis, Sharon Spencer, Phil Gamble, Michael Duffy, Joanne Clark
Illustrators	Mike Garland, Mark Walker, Darren R. Awuah, Debajyoti Dutta, Richard Tibbits, Phil Gamble, Peter Bull, Phil Wilson, Debbie Maizels
Production Editor	Nikoleta Parasaki
Production Controller	Mandy Inness
Cover Designer	Mark Cavanagh
Managing Editor	Stephanie Farrow
Managing Art Editor	Lee Griffiths

DK INDIA

Managing Editor	Pakshalika Jayaprakash
Senior Editor	Neha Gupta
Editor	Antara Moitra
Managing Art Editor	Arunesh Talapatra
Senior Art Editor	Anis Sayyed
Art Editors	Pooja Pipil, Supriya Mahajan, Swati Katyal
Assistant Art Editors	Aanchal Singal, Astha Singh, Namita, Niyati Gosain, Payal Rosalind Malik
DTP Manager	Balwant Singh
DTP Designer	Bimlesh Tiwary

First published in Great Britain in 2013
by Dorling Kindersley Limited
80 Strand, London WC2R 0RL

Penguin Group (UK)
10 9 8 7 6 5 4 3
022–184198–Jan/2013

Copyright © 2013 Dorling Kindersley Limited
All rights reserved.

No part of this publication may be reproduced,
stored in a retrieval system, or transmitted in any
form or by any means, electronic, mechanical,
photocopying, recording, or otherwise without the
prior written permission of the copyright owners.

A CIP catalogue record for this book is available
from the British Library.

ISBN 978-1-4093-7923-2

Printed and bound in China

**Discover more at
www.dk.com**

CONTENTS

1 INTRODUCTION

2 CORE-TRAINING EXERCISES

HOW TO USE THIS BOOK

Used together, the four sections of this book offer an integrated, user-friendly guide to core training. The introduction provides an excellent platform for the exercise section, which features a comprehensive range of stretches and core-training movements. The programmes and sports-specific sections then show you how to bring this knowledge together in your training.

INTRODUCTION

The book's introduction offers a clear and simple guide to the basics of core training. Beginning with a definition of what the core is, and how it works, the chapter explains how core strength helps with everyday activities, posture, sport, and pregnancy. With useful guidance on assessing and developing your core strength, it also provides essential advice on how to engage the key core muscles, and a range of suggested exercises to help with specific activities.

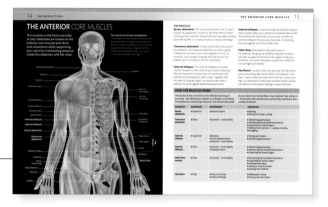

ANATOMICAL CORE DIAGRAMS
Detailed anatomical illustrations of your core muscles include details about the location and function of each and how they work together in body movements.

CORE-TRAINING EXERCISES

This section features over 150 exercises with additional variations and progressions to make each as versatile and as challenging as possible. The chapter's main four main sections (**»pp.56–165**) progress in order of increasing difficulty, and are bookended by a selection of mobility and static stretches (**»pp.44–55; 166–71**). The Visual Exercise Directory (**»pp.36–39**) at the start of the chapter enables you to navigate to individual exercises at a glance, while the Exercise Movement Matrix (**»pp.40–43**) groups each of the exercises by their Target Movement and Difficulty Rating to help with designing your own programmes (**»pp.186–89**). Each of the core-strength exercises featured in the main sections are accompanied by an information panel, which provides details of the Target Muscles, Target Movement, and Difficulty Rating of the exercise, along with an annotated anatomical artwork that shows you where each of the relevant muscles are located.

TARGET MUSCLES
Buttons on the panel show at a glance which core muscles the exercise works. Details of these 12 muscles and their function are provided in the Introduction (**»pp.14–17**).

DIFFICULTY RATING
The bar at the foot of the panel shows provides a score of 1–10 to give you an idea of how challenging each exercise is. Full details of this grading system are provided in the Introduction (**»p.31**).

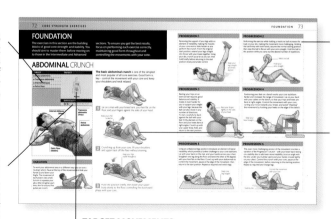

EXERCISE PROGRESSIONS
Increasingly difficult versions of key exercises are provided to challenge your core as your training progresses and your core strength, stability, and mobility improves.

STEP-BY-STEP SEQUENCES
User-friendly text and illustrations guide you through each of the exercises in a clear, straightforward way, with useful annotation to help you achieve the best possible form.

TARGET MOVEMENTS
The icon on the panel shows which of the six core movements are involved in the exercise – Isometric, Flexion, Extension, Side Flexion, Rotation, or Complex (**box opposite**).

TARGET MOVEMENT ICONS

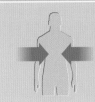

ISOMETRIC
Isometric strength is the ability to hold your body in a fixed position or resist an external force, such as when you are carrying a heavy weight.

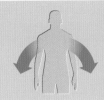

SIDE FLEXION
This movement involves bending from side to side from your waist or reaching overhead to either your left or your right.

FLEXION
Flexion involves bending forwards – for example, when you are picking something off the ground, or moving to sit or stand from a lying position.

ROTATION
Rotation involves turning movements from your waist, such as twisting to look over your shoulder.

EXTENSION
Extension involves bending your back to stand from a bent-over position, or arching your back to stretch up to reach something.

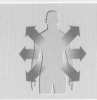

COMPLEX
Complex movements involve a combination of one or more of the other five movements listed in this table.

CORE-TRAINING PROGRAMMES

This chapter offers five easy-to-navigate three-part programmes to help you get the most out of your core training (**»pp.174–85**). There are also two handy tables to help you to create your own workouts (**»pp.186–89**), and a final programme you can use as a test or a fun challenge you can include in your training.

SPORTS-SPECIFIC CORE-TRAINING

This section profiles a comprehensive range of sports according to their principle core movements, with example exercises that may help to improve your performance. The table at the start of the chapter (**»pp.195–97**) offers a user-friendly reference to help you understand the key movements of your chosen sport.

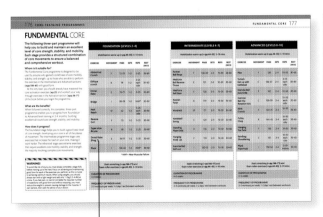

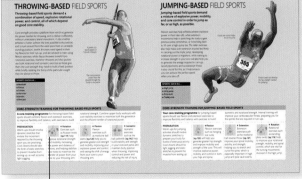

THREE-STAGE PROGRAMMES
Each of the easy-to-use programmes offer three levels of difficulty to help you progress in a safe and structured way and get the very best results from your training regimen.

SPORTS-SPECIFIC CORE MOVEMENTS
Information on the core movements for each group of sports helps you to gain a better understanding of how to train for your chosen activity.

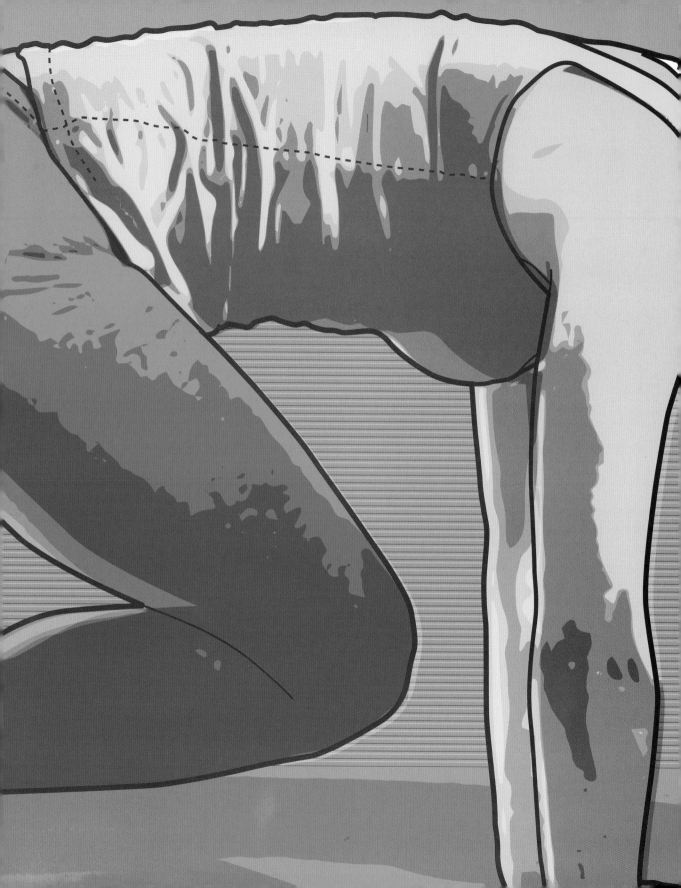

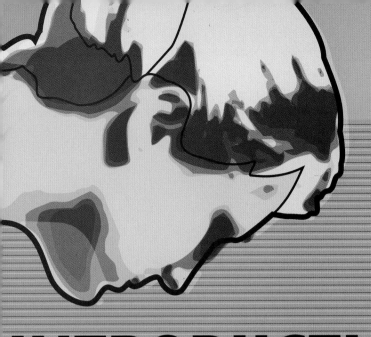

INTRODUCTION

1

WHAT IS THE CORE?

The core is the foundation for your movements, enabling mobility in the upper and lower body, directing power efficiently to your limbs, and stabilizing your spine, ribcage, and pelvis against the stress of those movements, or of external forces exterted upon them.

The core plays a key role in everyday biological functions. It creates internal pressure within the abdominal cavity, holding the internal organs in place, and helping with the expulsion of air from the lungs, and of bodily waste. The core muscles, in particular the transverse abdominis and pelvic floor (»p.15), are also active during childbirth.

AN INACTIVE CORE

Modern lifestyles are highly sedentary, meaning certain core muscles may become inactive. If you do not exercise your core muscles regularly, you will lose the ability to engage them instinctively while performing everyday movements such as bending and lifting. When this happens, other muscles may take over from them, which can lead to muscular imbalances – where one muscle is stronger than its opposing muscle – and, possibly, injury in the longer term. A common example of this is poor posture (»pp.32–33), which can cause imbalance in your hip and buttock muscles, resulting in lower-back pain. Core training helps to improve strength, stability, and mobility, reducing the likelihood of such imbalances developing.

THE KINETIC CHAIN

The kinetic chain is a movement system consisting of myofascial (muscular), articular (joints), and neural (motor) components. Each of these individual elements are dependent on the others for optimum performance, both when the body is moving and when it is stationary but active – for example when you are holding a weight in your arms.

The idea behind the kinetic chain, as demonstrated in the illustrations shown here, is that every part of your body, including muscles, joints, and nerves, must work together to produce movements. It is particularly important to keep this in mind when bending and lifting, exercising, and playing sport to ensure you are using the right muscles in the right way, thus reducing the possibility of muscular imbalance and injury.

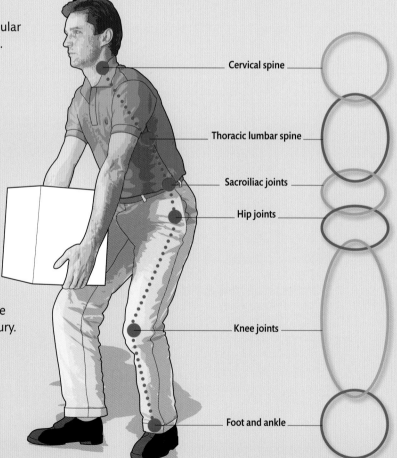

Cervical spine

Thoracic lumbar spine

Sacroiliac joints

Hip joints

Knee joints

Foot and ankle

Everyday activities
Something as simple as lifting a box sets off a chain of movement running through the body. Movement produced at any joint in the kinetic chain directly affects the joints above and below it.

THE IMPORTANCE OF THE CORE

Your core acts as an axis along which the muscles of the hips, abdomen, and back interact to support and stabilize the spine, providing a solid base for movement in the legs and arms. It is a key part of your body's support structure – if you were to strip the spine of all muscle, leaving just bones and ligaments, it would collapse under 9kg (20lb) of load. Strong core muscles generate the strength, stability, and mobility needed to carry out everyday activities such as carrying shopping, climbing the stairs, and getting into a car. They also play a crucial role in more demanding dynamic sports, helping to transmit increased power and stability, and performance, while also reducing the risk of sustaining injury. As a result, core development is a key objective of elite athletes and their coaches.

FUNCTIONS OF THE CORE

Although traditionally associated with the abdomen, the core plays an important role in functions throughout the body:
- Stabilizing the thoracic cage and pelvis during movement
- Providing internal pressure for biological functions
- Maintaining the strength, stability, and mobility of the spine
- Providing an axis of power for the kinetic chain (**below**)

BENEFITS OF CORE TRAINING

A balanced and focused core-training programme can have a positive impact on your physical wellbeing as a whole. The benefits of core training include:
- Improved posture
- Increased protection and "bracing" of your back
- Greater balance and co-ordination
- Greater power and speed

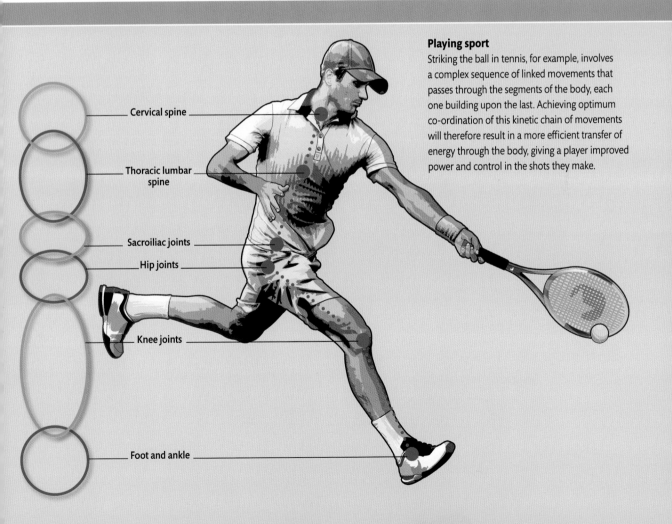

Cervical spine

Thoracic lumbar spine

Sacroiliac joints

Hip joints

Knee joints

Foot and ankle

Playing sport
Striking the ball in tennis, for example, involves a complex sequence of linked movements that passes through the segments of the body, each one building upon the last. Achieving optimum co-ordination of this kinetic chain of movements will therefore result in a more efficient transfer of energy through the body, giving a player improved power and control in the shots they make.

SPINE

is the central support
your entire body, assisting
all movement, while
and protecting your
. It must be firm enough
ur body weight when
et flexible and strong
anchor your body and
upper and lower
ove smoothly.

The regions of the spine

The spine is a column of up to 33 bones called
vertebrae. All but nine of these vertebrae are movable
and they are divided into three groups: cervical (neck),
thoracic (mid-back), and lumbar (lower back). The
remaining nine vertebrae are located at the base of the
spine, fused together to form the sacrum (hip complex).

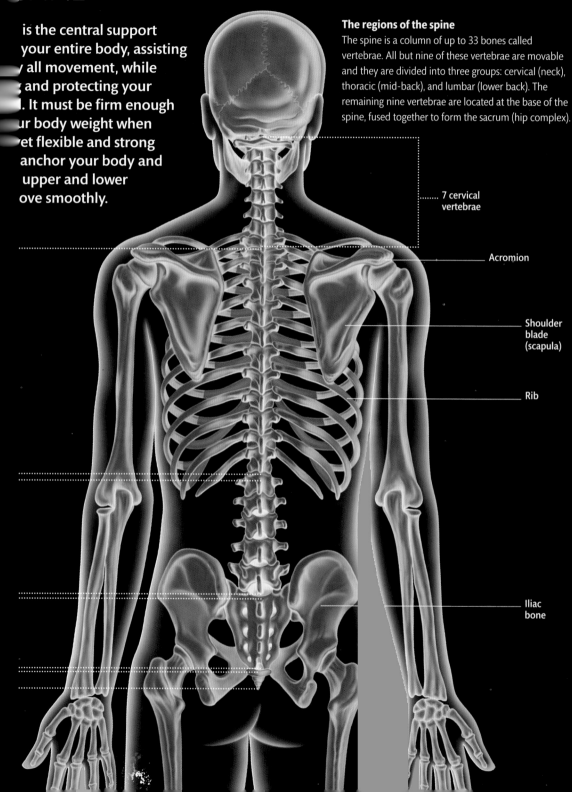

7 cervical
vertebrae

Acromion

Shoulder
blade
(scapula)

Rib

Iliac
bone

HOW THE SPINE WORKS

To understand how the spine supports the body and controls movement, it is helpful to divide it into four main sections – the neck (cervical), mid-back (thoracic), lower back (lumbar), and hip complex (sacrum). Individually, these perform different primary functions, such as controlling movement of the head; together they bring about movements that involve the whole body.

Movement of the spine

There is very little movement between adjacent vertebrae of the spine. However, the combined movement of vertebrae along the length of the spine enables considerable total body movement.

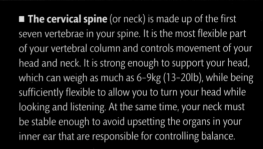

7 cervical vertebrae

12 thoracic vertebrae

5 lumbar vertebrae

Sacrum

■ **The cervical spine** (or neck) is made up of the first seven vertebrae in your spine. It is the most flexible part of your vertebral column and controls movement of your head and neck. It is strong enough to support your head, which can weigh as much as 6–9kg (13–20lb), while being sufficiently flexible to allow you to turn your head while looking and listening. At the same time, your neck must be stable enough to avoid upsetting the organs in your inner ear that are responsible for controlling balance.

■ **The thoracic spine** (or mid-back) is the longest portion of your spinal column and is made up of the middle 12 vertebrae. The primary function of your thoracic spine is to protect the organs in the chest cavity by holding your ribcage in place. Although the ribcage's bulk provides protection, it also greatly restricts the amount of movement possible in your thorax. As a result, movement of your mid-back is mostly restricted to rotation – when you twist your upper body, it rotates around the thoracic spine – and a small amount of flexion and extension.

■ **The lumbar spine** (or lower back) is a more mobile part of your vertebral column. It consists of five vertebrae and sits immediately below your thoracic spine. You use this section of the spine for many basic activities, such as bending forwards, walking, and running. Connected to your pelvis, which is relatively immobile, this area is key to generating the power of core movements and bears most of the weight when your body is upright.

■ **The sacrum** (or hip complex) is made up of five fused – and therefore relatively immobile – sacral vertebrae that are important for stabilizing the other bones and muscles of your pelvis and hips. The sacrum is noticeably different in men and women, with the bone being longer and narrower in men than it is in women. The sacral vertebrae are connected to the vertebrae at the end of your spine – known as the coccygeal vertebrae – by a joint called the sacrococcygeal symphysis. Together, the coccygeal vertebrae form the coccyx, or tailbone.

THE ANTERIOR CORE MUSCLES

The muscles to the front and sides of your abdomen are known as the anterior core muscles and drive core movement while supporting your spine by maintaining pressure inside the abdomen and the chest.

The muscles of the hips and abdomen
The anterior core muscles work with those of the back and buttocks in supporting and stabilizing the spine, and are important in driving rotational movement and hip flexion. Together with the lumbar region of the back, these muscles play a vital role in building core strength.

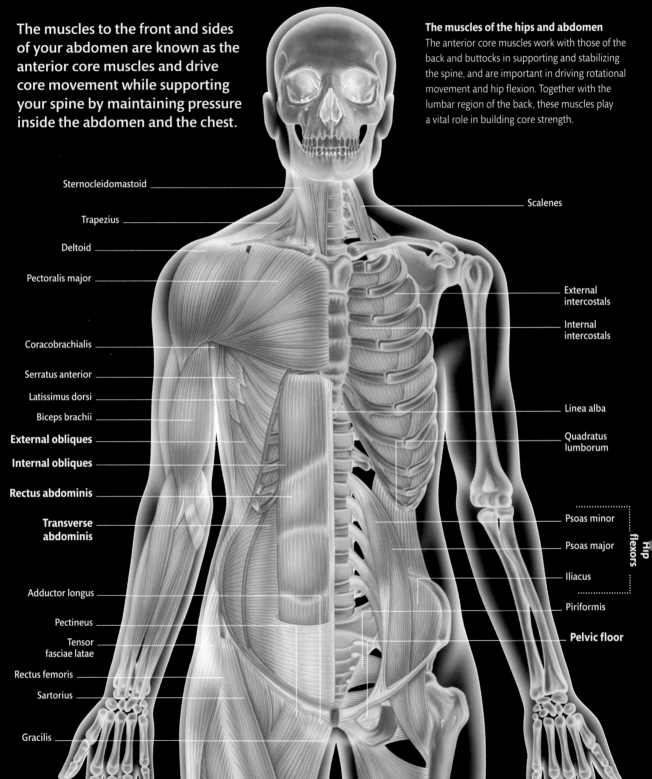

Sternocleidomastoid
Trapezius
Deltoid
Pectoralis major
Coracobrachialis
Serratus anterior
Latissimus dorsi
Biceps brachii
External obliques
Internal obliques
Rectus abdominis
Transverse abdominis
Adductor longus
Pectineus
Tensor fasciae latae
Rectus femoris
Sartorius
Gracilis

Scalenes
External intercostals
Internal intercostals
Linea alba
Quadratus lumborum
Psoas minor
Psoas major
Iliacus
Piriformis
Pelvic floor

Hip flexors

THE MUSCLES

Rectus abdominis The rectus abdominis is the "six-pack" muscle, its appearance caused by the three fibrous bands running across it and the vertical band (the linea alba) running down the middle. It is mainly involved in flexion (bending).

Transverse abdominis A deep muscle that runs around the abdomen, the transverse abdominis acts like a girdle, holding the muscles of your core together. It is key to isometric core strength (resisting external forces) and stability, and is involved in all core movements.

External obliques The external obliques are surface muscles located on either side of your rectus abdominis. They are important to rotational core movements and side flexion (bending from side to side). Together with the internal obliques (**right**), the muscles also help to stabilize the spine against lateral (sideways) forces.

Internal obliques Located beneath the external obliques, these muscles help you to perform movements that involve the rotation and side flexion of your core. As with the external obliques they are also important in stabilizing the spine against forces from either side.

Pelvic floor Running from the pubic bone to the tailbone, this group of small but important muscles provides a support structure for the organs inside your abdomen. As a result, they play a crucial role in effective core strength and stability.

Hip flexors Located within the hip joint, the hip flexors (psoas muscle group) control flexion movements in the hips – that is, when you bend from the hip or raise your legs. It is important to keep these muscles mobile, as they can often be overworked, leading to lower-back pain.

HOW THE MUSCLES WORK

The muscles of your core are key to the efficient functioning of your body – they affect posture, balance, co-ordination, and mobility, and stabilize your trunk during movements. This table provides details of your anterior core muscles (those of your abdomen, hips, and groin) – their location, their main functions, and how they contribute to basic everyday movements.

MUSCLES	LOCATION	MOVEMENT	FUNCTION
Rectus abdominis	■ Superficial	■ Flexion of spine	■ Bending ■ Moving from lying to sitting
Transverse abdominis	■ Deep	■ Isometric – trunk stability	■ Maintaining good posture ■ Maintaining internal abdominal pressure ■ Supporting the internal organs ■ Helping forced expiration – coughing, sneezing, and laughing
External obliques	■ Superficial	■ Rotation ■ Some sideways flexion ■ Isometric – trunk stability	■ Twisting and rotation ■ Maintaining good posture
Internal obliques	■ Deep	■ Isometric – trunk stability ■ Sideways flexion	■ Maintaining good posture ■ Maintaining internal abdominal pressure ■ Supporting the internal organs
Pelvic floor muscles	■ Deep	■ Isometric – trunk stability	■ Maintaining internal abdominal pressure ■ Supporting the internal organs ■ Assisting when lifting ■ Helping to control urination ■ Assisting with childbirth
Hip flexors	■ Deep	■ Flexion of the hip ■ Lifting of the legs	■ Walking and running ■ Going up and down stairs

THE POSTERIOR CORE MUSCLES

The core muscles of the back (posterior core muscles) are built up in layers around the skeleton. These muscles provide strength, support, and stability to your spine, and drive hip movement.

The muscles of the back and buttocks
The posterior core muscles work with those of the abdomen and hips in supporting and stabilizing the spine against external movements, and controlling most of the movements of the hip joint.

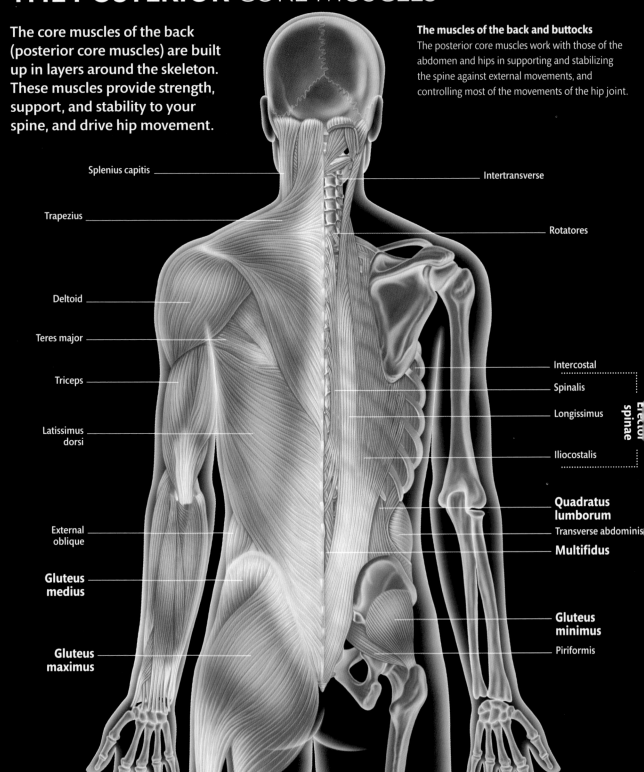

Splenius capitis

Trapezius

Deltoid

Teres major

Triceps

Latissimus dorsi

External oblique

Gluteus medius

Gluteus maximus

Intertransverse

Rotatores

Intercostal

Spinalis

Longissimus

Iliocostalis

Erector spinae

Quadratus lumborum

Transverse abdominis

Multifidus

Gluteus minimus

Piriformis

THE MUSCLES

Erector spinae The erector spinae (spinal erectors) are a group of long tendinous muscles that run the length of the spine. They provide support to your spine when you flex it (bend forwards) and extend it (bend backwards), and are also involved in stabilizing it against sideways movement.

Multifidus The multifidus is a series of muscles attached to the spine, which work to keep it straight and stabilized while helping to distribute body weight evenly along it. They also play a protective role, stiffening the spine to resist forces that might cause it to bend.

Quadratus lumborum The inner portion of the quadratus lumborum is adjacent to the spine and counters any sideways force, such as that caused by holding a suitcase or shopping bag in one hand.

Gluteus minimus The smallest of the muscles in the buttocks, the gluteus minimus lies beneath the gluteus medius, with which it works to abduct the thigh (lift it outwards). It is also involved in hip rotation and helps to hold the pelvis in a stable position.

Gluteus medius The second-largest muscle in the buttocks, the gluteus medius lies between the gluteus minimus and maximus. It assists with hip abduction and rotation, whilst also providing stability to the pelvic region.

Gluteus maximus The largest and most superficial of the three gluteal muscles, the gluteus maximus gives the buttocks their shape and appearance. It is involved in hip abduction, rotation, and extension, while also stabilizing the whole of the pelvic area.

HOW THE MUSCLES WORK

The muscles of your back and buttocks play a key role in core strength. Your back muscles affect posture, balance, co-ordination, and mobility, and stabilize your trunk during movements. This table provides details of the posterior core muscles found in your lower back and buttocks – their location, their main functions, and how they contribute to everyday movements.

MUSCLES	LOCATION	MOVEMENT	FUNCTION
Erector spinae	■ Deep	■ Extension ■ Provides support during flexion ■ Support and straightening of the spine	■ Bending forwards and backwards ■ Maintaining good posture
Multifidus	■ Deep	■ Extension ■ Sideways flexion ■ Isometric – trunk stability	■ Maintaining good posture ■ Stiffening the spine to resist bending forces
Quadratus lumborum	■ Deep	■ Sideways flexion	■ Stabilizing the spine against lateral movement ■ Lifting heavy objects ■ Carrying a suitcase
Gluteus minimus	■ Deep	■ Hip abduction ■ Transverse hip abduction ■ Internal hip rotation	■ Getting out of a car
Gluteus medius	■ Deep	■ Hip abduction ■ Transverse hip abduction ■ Internal hip rotation ■ External hip rotation (during hip abduction)	■ Stepping sideways
Gluteus maximus	■ Superficial	■ Hip abduction ■ Hip extension ■ External hip rotation	■ Walking ■ Running ■ Jumping ■ Cycling ■ Going up and down stairs

WHAT IS CORE TRAINING?

Core training focuses on three areas: core mobility, core stability, and core strength. Each of these plays an important role in the health, support, and function of your body, and so achieving a balance between them is vital. The starting point of this process lies in learning how to activate, strengthen, and control the muscles of your pelvic floor.

WHAT IS CORE MOBILITY?

Core mobility refers to the movement of your spine and hips. There are five main movement patterns involved: isometric, flexion, extension, side flexion, and rotation. It is vital to mobilize your spine and hips before exercise, to loosen tight muscles and encourage weaker, under-used muscles to function correctly. This helps to balance the relationship between muscle length and movement patterns, and allows for deeper muscle activation, improving your core stability and strength. It is best to maintain a full, natural range of motion to keep your body functioning properly. Joints and muscles that are hypomobile (stiff) or hypermobile (too mobile) will inevitably lead to imbalances. When this happens, one area of the body is forced to compensate for the lack, or increased range, of movement in another – increasing your chances of injury.

WHAT IS CORE STABILITY?

Core stability is the ability to control the position and movement of your mid-section (trunk), in order to improve your posture and improve the efficiency of your limb movement. Core-stability training targets the deep muscles of your abdomen, hips, and spine to create a base for support. The main deep muscles are the multifidus, transverse abdominis, and pelvic floor, which form a "cylinder" around the lower torso, with the transverse abdominis to the front, the multifidus to the back, and the pelvic floor forming the base. During most types of body movement – lifting, bending, sitting, twisting, walking, running, or jumping – these three muscles work to stabilize your lumbar spine, while your gluteus and quadratus lumborum muscles work to stabilize your pelvis.

The stability of your back depends on all of these muscles being strong and working together effectively. Because of the complex network of muscles and fascia (connective tissues) involved in this structure, activating or "waking up" your core is a key part of training. You may find it hard to activate the deeper core muscles to start with, so you should begin by following the basic exercises in Activating Your Core (**»p.25**), before you move on to those in the Activation section of Core-Training Exercises (**»pp.56–71**).

WHAT IS CORE STRENGTH?

Core strength is the ability to perform challenging physical tasks that demand good form and control. As it involves all of the muscles of your core – both deep and superficial – it has a key role in core training, but it is important to remember that good core strength requires a foundation of good core stability first. Core-strength training works by pushing your core muscles beyond their normal demands or by holding positions to increase endurance strength. The greater the force exerted upon the body, the greater the amount of core muscle engagement, and thus the degree of core muscle activation and strength required. As you develop core strength through exercise, your movements will become adapted to a higher level of skill and performance.

CORE TRAINING AND THE PELVIC FLOOR

The pelvic floor is the group of muscles and fascia that form the base of your abdominal cylinder. These muscles and fascia have a number of functions – holding your pelvis together; maintaining the position of the pelvic organs, and supporting them against gravity; and helping to control the flow of urine from your bladder and waste from your rectum. Poor physical fitness, as well as pregnancy, ageing, and injury, can cause a weakening of the muscles in this area, so it is important to keep them as strong as possible.

These muscles also play a key role in effective core strength because they help to activate the transverse abdominis, along with the other stabilizing muscles of your core. It is therefore important to learn how to control and activate your pelvic floor muscles (**»p.25**), possibly with Kegel exercises (the conscious engagement and contraction of your pelvic floor muscles), before attempting any of the movements in the exercise sections (**»pp.34–171**).

CORE TRAINING – KEY AREAS

Although different activities make different demands on your core, an overall core workout should focus on three primary areas: mobility, stability, and strength. Where possible, you should try to develop a training programme that combines these with the five main types of core-based movement – isometric, flexion, extension, side flexion, and rotation – see Core-Training Programmes (**»pp.172–91**).

MOBILITY

- Encourages natural range of movement and increases flexibility
- Balances the muscle lengths between antagonistic muscles groups
- Promotes relaxation and tension relief
- Aligns the body and improves posture
- Improves efficiency of muscle activation and reactivity
- Increases stability and strength
- Decreases the risk of pain and injury
- Good core mobility exercises include:

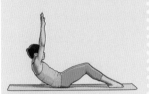

Roll-back
- (**»p.90**)

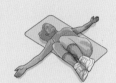

Hip roll
- (**»pp.88–89**)

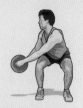

Medicine ball chop
- (**»pp.136**)

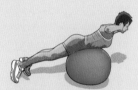

Exercise ball back extension
- (**»p.122**)

STABILITY

- Improves posture and skeletal alignment
- Helps prevent pain and injury
- Increases body awareness, control, and balance
- Resists unwanted movement of the spine
- Provides the stability and support for daily tasks
- Helps to build muscle strength and improve limb movement
- Improves performance in sporting activity
- Good core stability exercises include:

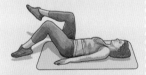

Toe tap
- (**»pp.62–63**)

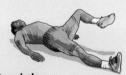

Leg circle
- (**»p.74**)

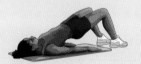

Bridge
- (**»pp.98–99**)

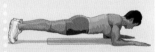

Plank
- (**»pp.102–03**)

STRENGTH

- Enhances all-round body strength and function
- Makes it easier to perform a range of everyday tasks
- Improves balance and control
- Increases speed and agility
- Helps to enhance power of your movements
- Improves performance in sporting activity
- Creates lean muscle tone
- Good core strength exercises include:

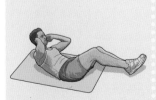

V leg-raise
- (**»p.92**)

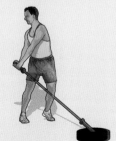

O-bar rotation
- (**»pp.114–15**)

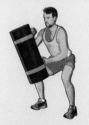

Sandbag shouldering
- (**»p.151**)

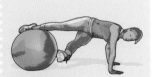

Exercise ball hip rotation kick
- (**»pp.158–59**)

CORE TRAINING AND EVERYDAY ACTIVITIES

Every day, you perform numerous core-related movements. In addition to obvious activities like exercise or sport, work-based tasks and chores, such as sitting at a desk or carrying bags, all place demands on your core. Building and maintaining good core strength is therefore essential.

Learning correct postural alignment and how to stabilize your spine can help to ease the strain of everyday activities, prevent pain and injury, and make you feel stronger and more confident. Whether you are digging in the garden, lifting heavy objects, or carrying your child, it is the strength from the deep centring muscles of your abdomen and lower back (lumbar spine) that will enable you to perform these tasks safely.

THE BODY'S "POWERHOUSE"

Your core is often referred to as the body's "powerhouse", a central region providing a girdle of strength and connecting the abdomen with the lower back and hips. The abdominal area, in conjunction with the deep spinal muscles, create a stable base for generating strength and providing support for all movement. As a result it is important to understand the concepts behind core strength and train correctly. Pushing your body too far or too fast, without the support of your core, can lead to you using the wrong muscles and ingraining poor movement patterns, which, over time, may lead to muscular imbalance, reduced power and possibly even injury. However, while it is important to practise core activation, constantly holding your deep abdominals in a braced contraction may potentially interfere with the pump-like motion of your diaphragm, restricting the efficiency of your breathing. You should therefore look to engage your core as part of a fitness programme, or before attempting to lift a load, rather than on a moment-to-moment basis.

Many of us are not used to training the deep muscles of the core, often focusing instead on the more visible outer muscles of the torso such as the rectus abdominus. These large muscles, known as primary movers, can be felt when performing everyday activities and training for fitness. Due to their size and power they can often take over the work of the stabilizing muscles, leaving the body less supported and vulnerable to strain. For this reason, a balanced and comprehensive approach to core training is vital.

CORE STRENGTH AND EVERYDAY ACTIVITIES

Sitting at your desk
■ **Core strength benefits**
▶ Stability in lumbar spine ▶ Mobility in back, shoulders, and hips ▶ Strong sitting posture
▶ Reduced lower back tension, hunched shoulders, and tightness in hip flexors
▶ Reduced risk of back pain and injury
■ **Core exercises that can help**
▶ Back extension (**»p.69**)
▶ Oyster (**»p.66**)
▶ Leg circle (**»p.74**)

Using a phone
■ **Core strength benefits**
▶ Mobility in neck and shoulders ▶ Stability in upper body and shoulders ▶ Strong postural muscles ▶ Good sitting posture ▶ Reduced risk of neck and back pain and injury
■ **Core exercises that can help**
▶ Dart (**»p.65**)
▶ Dorsal raise (**»pp.76–77**)
▶ Superman (**»pp.70–71**)

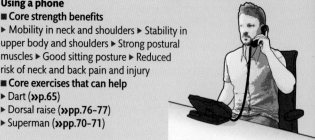

Lifting
■ **Core strength benefits**
▶ Mobility in neck and shoulder ▶ Stability in upper back and shoulders ▶ Strong postural muscles ▶ Isometric strength ▶ Good lifting technique ▶ Reduced risk of back pain and injury
■ **Core exercises that can help**
▶ Superman (**»pp.70–71**)
▶ Dorsal raise (**»pp.76–77**)
▶ Double leg lower and lift (**»pp.100–01**)

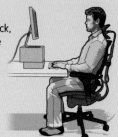

Carrying bags (laptop or handbag)
■ **Core strength benefits**
▶ Isometric strength ▶ Spinal stability against lateral (sideways) forces ▶ Strong postural muscles
▶ Strong, balanced posture ▶ Reduced shoulder muscle tightness ▶ Reduced risk of injury
■ **Core exercises that can help**
▶ Swim (**»p.94**)
▶ Hip roll (**»pp.88–89**)
▶ Side bend (**»p.81**)

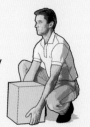

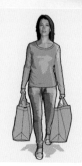

EXERCISES FOR EVERYDAY ACTIVITIES

Listed below is a selection of exercises that will help you to strengthen, stabilize, and mobilize your core, and assist with a wide range of everyday activities. It is important to train your core properly to maintain good movement and reduce the risk of sustaining injury.

EXERCISE	BENEFITS	EXERCISE	BENEFITS
Active pelvic floor (»p.56)	■ Activation of deep abdominals. Improves posture; helps with lifting and carrying.	**Leg circle** (»p.74)	■ Hip and lumbar stability. Helps with sideways movement, and lifting uneven loads.
Pillow squeeze (»p.58)	■ Hip stability. Aids lateral (sideways) movements, such as getting in and out of a car.	**Dorsal raise** (»p.76)	■ Thoracic mobility and strength; shoulder alignment. Improves posture.
Oyster (»p.66)	■ Hip stability. Assists lateral movements, such as getting in and out of a car.	**Side-lying leg lift** (»pp.84–85)	■ Spinal alignment; hip and lumbar stability and strength. Assists lifting and carrying.
Dart (»p.65)	■ Spinal and shoulder alignment. Improves posture; helps with lifting and carrying.	**Hip roll** (»p.88)	■ Lumbar rotation, mobility, stability, and strength. Improving seated posture.
Toe tap (»p.62)	■ Lumbar and thoracic stability. Helps with lifting and maintaining good posture.	**Roll-back** (»p.90)	■ Mobility and strength in muscles of spine, deep core, and hip flexors. Aids posture.
Prone leg lift (»p.67)	■ Glute and hamstring strength. Improves posture; can ease lumbar pain from sitting.	**Swim** (»p.94)	■ Spinal stability and strength. Assists with lifting and carrying uneven loads.
Star (»p.68)	■ Spinal stability; hip and shoulder alignment. Aids posture, and lifting and carrying.	**Bridge** (»p.98)	■ Hip and spinal mobility and strength. Aids sideways movements, and lifting and carrying.
Abdominal crunch (»p.72)	■ Cervical and thoracic mobility and strength. Assists bending and climbing the stairs.	**Plank** (»p.102)	■ Spinal alignment and strength. Improves posture; helps with lifting and carrying.

Lifting your baby
■ **Core strength benefits**
▶ Strong postural muscles ▶ Stability in lumbar spine against lateral (sideways) and rotational forces ▶ Lateral, rotational, and isometric strength ▶ Good posture ▶ Reduced lower back tension, and risk of injury
■ **Core exercises that can help**
▶ Star (»p.68)
▶ Super-slow bicycle (»p.95)
▶ Bridge (»p.98)

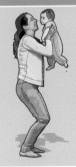

Doing housework
■ **Core strength benefits**
▶ Stability and strength in all movements
▶ Stability in upper back and lumbar spine against lateral (sideways) and rotational forces
▶ Reduced lower back pain and stiff shoulders, and risk of injury
■ **Core exercises that can help**
▶ Oblique reach (»pp.86–87)
▶ Dart (»p.65)
▶ Side-lying leg lift (»pp.84–85)

Gardening
■ **Core strength benefits**
▶ Spinal mobility ▶ Isometric, lateral (sideways), and rotational strength ▶ Spinal stability against lateral and rotational forces ▶ Reduced tension in lower back and shoulders
■ **Core exercises that can help**
▶ Oblique crunch (»p.79)
▶ Back extension (»p.69)
▶ Plank (»pp.102–03)

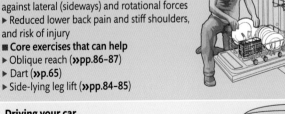

Driving your car
■ **Core strength benefits**
▶ Mobility in neck, shoulders, and lumbar spine ▶ Lumbar stability and strength
▶ Isometric and extension strengt
▶ Strong posture ▶ Reduced lower back, shoulders, and hip flexor pain
■ **Core exercises that can help**
▶ Dorsal raise (»pp.76–77)
▶ Oyster (»p.66)
▶ Horizontal balance (»p.97)

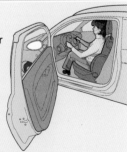

CORE TRAINING AND POSTURE

The lumbar region is crucial in developing core strength. Consequently, it is important to keep your lower back healthy by maintaining good posture. The best posture for you is the one in which your back is put under the least strain. Whether you are standing or sitting, the muscles in your back should be relaxed without being slack, and your spine should be gently S-shaped.

GOOD POSTURE

The way you stand and hold yourself makes a big difference to the way you look and feel. A "good" standing posture is one in which your body looks symmetrical – equally aligned from side to side and back to front (**near and far right**). This position puts less stress on your spine, minimizing wear and tear, and reducing the risk of injury.

The key to good posture lies in developing and maintaining a combination of good core strength and general fitness. Core-strength training gives you a feel for the way your body works – particularly the natural patterns of movement. General fitness helps you to maintain a healthy weight, reducing stress on your weight-bearing muscles and joints. It also promotes mental and emotional balance, making you less likely to tense your muscles, further benefiting your posture.

BAD POSTURE

Although "bad" posture is generally used to mean slack posture, an excessively rigid body position can be equally bad for you (**middle right**). In reality, bad posture is generally classed as anything which puts your spine under unnecessary strain, resulting in tension in the back and placing stress on the muscles, ligaments, discs, and spinal joints.

THE CAUSES OF BAD POSTURE

Whether you are standing, sitting, or performing movements of any kind, your muscular system tends to take the path of least resistance with regards to posture. If you are fit and your body is functioning properly and efficiently, this should not cause problems. However, poor posture can occur if certain muscles or muscle groups are overactive, underactive, or imbalanced. Causes of these problems include a lack of

mobility; poor technique when exercising or performing everyday tasks; and the effect of gravity on your spine over time.

If the natural movement patterns of your hips and spine are restricted – if you work at a desk, for example – imbalances can occur in your muscles, causing bad posture, and possibly back pain and injury. To combat this take regular breaks from your desk, and use stretches to keep your muscles and joints mobile. Exercising or performing household tasks with poor or incorrect technique can also result in bad posture, because you are engaging the wrong muscles at the expense of the right ones. Being more aware of your movements will allow you to move in the right way, as well as identifying the source of any problems.

STANDING POSTURE

Posture has a direct impact on joints and muscles. Aim for a balanced upright posture, with your body weight evenly distributed from front to back.

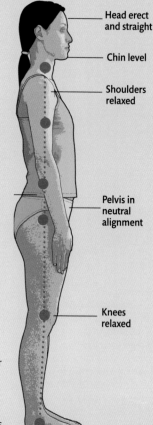

Head erect and straight

Chin level

Shoulders relaxed

Gentle S-curve in spine

Pelvis in neutral alignment

Knees relaxed

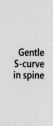 **Correct pelvic angle**
It may take some time to get this stance right, but the trick is to remember to tuck in your pelvis. This involves consciously tilting your pelvis into a neutral alignment so your lower back has a slight curve, rather than an unnatural, hollowed-out appearance that puts the lower back under stress.

The day-to-day compressional pressure of gravity on your spine can affect posture in the long term, which is why it is important to use your core to stand tall and sit up straight.

GOOD SITTING POSTURE

Sitting for prolonged periods of time can trigger pain in your lower back because sitting places a greater strain on your spine than standing or walking. Adopting a good sitting position is not difficult and will reduce the stress you place on your back.

A good sitting position does not require you to sit up straight for long periods – you must relax in order to avoid straining your muscles. Anyone attempting to sit bolt upright will gradually slip into a relaxed, slouched position. Practitioners of postural education methods such as the Alexander Technique encourage people to find just the right amount of curve in their neck, mid-back, and lower back.

If you use a desk for long periods of time, sit in a well-designed chair, set up your workstation to avoid stretching or straining, and try to take regular breaks. At home, choose a comfortable chair with enough space to let you change your position and move around while watching television or reading. You can also place cushions behind your lower back to support your spine.

BAD SITTING POSTURE

Many of us spend our days sitting at a desk so it is important to get into the habit of maintaining good posture. Slouching – with your shoulders and pelvis pushed forwards – is one of the most common forms of poor sitting position. It causes problems throughout the body ranging from backache to musculoskeletal pains, joint pains, and tension headaches. Slouching forwards also compresses your diaphragm, resulting in restricted breathing.

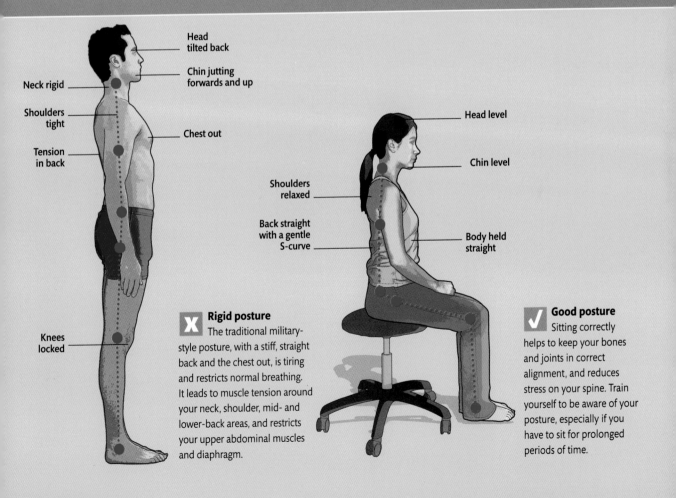

Head tilted back

Chin jutting forwards and up

Neck rigid

Shoulders tight

Tension in back

Chest out

Knees locked

X **Rigid posture**
The traditional military-style posture, with a stiff, straight back and the chest out, is tiring and restricts normal breathing. It leads to muscle tension around your neck, shoulder, mid- and lower-back areas, and restricts your upper abdominal muscles and diaphragm.

Head level

Chin level

Shoulders relaxed

Back straight with a gentle S-curve

Body held straight

✓ **Good posture**
Sitting correctly helps to keep your bones and joints in correct alignment, and reduces stress on your spine. Train yourself to be aware of your posture, especially if you have to sit for prolonged periods of time.

THE IMPORTANCE OF CORRECT HIP PLACEMENT

The pelvis is the key weight-bearing centre of your body. Not only does it support your spine and head but it is also the vital link between your upper body and your legs. Any movements you make with your pelvis trigger movements in your spine: tilting your pelvis backwards and forwards creates spinal flexion and extension, while moving from side to side and twisting causes side flexion and spinal rotation. Establishing and maintaining correct hip placement are therefore important to the alignment of your spine as well as to your overall core strength. Most everyday activities and sports involve a combination of movements across the body and maintaining correct hip placement will enable you to perform these with good posture and form, thus reducing pressure on your spine and your risk of injury.

NEUTRAL HIP AND SPINAL ALIGNMENT

When your pelvis is in a "neutral" position, the front hip bones are horizontally aligned to one another and vertically aligned with the pubic bone, so the pelvis should neither be tilted forward, backward, or rotated. This is the most even balanced position for the pelvis, in relation to your spine and thigh bones, providing a stable base for your body to move. This is therefore an ideal starting position for most movements that will encouraging correct spinal alignment and balance the joints and muscles that support it.

POSTURAL PROBLEMS

Acquired and genetic conditions can alter the shape of the spine, resulting in impaired movement and pain. Building your core strength can limit the impact of these problems, improving your balance and posture, or prevent them occurring in the first place.

Head tilted forwards and down

Chin low

Neck flexed

Shoulders hunched (lordosis)

Chest sagging

Exaggerated curve in spine (kyphosis)

Pelvis tilted forwards

Knees locked

Lordosis and kyphosis

Here, the head and chin hang low, the neck sticks forwards, and the upper back and shoulders are rounded and hunched. The muscles supporting the spinal column and abdomen are slack, and the pelvis is tilted forwards, which produces an overly hollowed-out back.

■ **Lordosis** (or sway back) is a common postural problem that occurs when the lumbar curve becomes over-pronounced. Viewed from the side, this means the belly tends to stick out to the front and the buttocks to the rear. Often occurring in conjunction with kyphosis (below), it can be caused by poor core stability, or tight hip flexor muscles and weak back muscles. The condition can be treated with corrective exercises, but left untreated, it can cause lower-back pain and disc problems.

■ **Kyphosis** is a spinal curvature leading to the rounding of the back. Often linked with lordosis (above) it is sometimes caused by over-shortened chest muscles pulling on the shoulder girdle. In mild cases, it appears as a slouching posture; in extreme cases it can leave sufferers with severe hunching. Most cases only require routine monitoring but serious ones can be debilitating, or even life threatening, due to the pressure placed on internal organs.

■ **Scoliosis** (right) is a curvature of the spine to one side. The condition often begins in childhood and can be mild, with few or no symptoms. Severe cases, however, can cause problems with posture, breathing, and walking. Obvious signs of the condition might include uneven shoulders, a tendency to lean to one side, or one prominent shoulder blade.

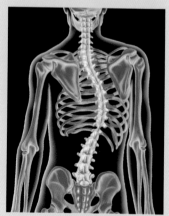

ACTIVATING YOUR CORE

Learning how to achieve a neutral hip and spinal alignment, and to engage or "switch on" the muscles of your core are crucial first steps to developing a strong and stable foundation for core training. Engaging your core effectively means activating and controlling the muscles that make up your "abdominal cylinder". The two key muscles to learn to control are your pelvic floor and your tranverse abdominis.

ACHIEVING NEUTRAL PELVIS AND SPINAL ALIGNMENT

The pelvis is the base support of your body and supports your spine. For optimum movement your pelvis should be in a "neutral" position – that is the most balanced position possible. A neutral pelvis will help to align your spine, improve posture, and provide a stable platform for all of your body's movements.

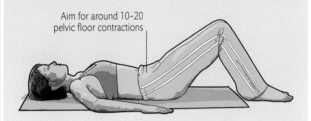

Place your hands in a triangle

Lie on your back with your hands on your lower stomach, making a triangle with your thumbs and index fingers. Allow your weight to press down through your tailbone. When your pelvis is in neutral, your hands will be level and your lumbar spine in a neutral curve.

ACTIVATING YOUR PELVIC FLOOR MUSCLES

Your pelvic floor muscles form the base of your abdominal cylinder. In addition to their primary role in controlling the passing of urine and faeces from your body, they also help you to activate your transverse abdominis and other core stabilizers. Learning to control these muscles is therefore key to core strength.

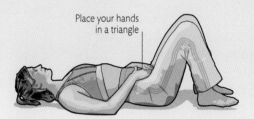

Aim for around 10–20 pelvic floor contractions

Lie on your back with your spine in a neutral position. Gently press the small of your back into the floor and tilt your pubic bone upwards. Contract the muscles that help you control the flow of passing urine. Repeatedly tense and release these muscles 10–20 times then relax.

LOCATING YOUR TRANSVERSE ABDOMINIS

Your transverse abdominis muscle is the deepest layer of your abdominals. Wrapping around your midsection like a corset, it forms the front wall of of your abdominal cylinder, stabilizing your lower back and pulling in the lower abdominal wall. Learning to activate and control your transverse abdominis is a vital component of good core strength. The first step in this process is to learn how to locate, or feel, where it is.

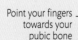

Point your fingers towards your pubic bone

Stand up straight with your back in a neutral position, with your hands forming a triangle over the front of your pelvis. Cough strongly. You will feel your transverse abdominis move beneath your fingers. Next, breath in and out. You will feel the muscle contract as you do so.

ACTIVATING YOUR TRANSVERSE ABDOMINIS

Once you have located your transverse abdominis muscles (**left**), the next stage involves learning to activate and control it, in order to give you a good base for all other core strength exercises. The key is to focus on drawing your navel towards your spine, hollowing your stomach, and tightening your waistline. You should aim to contract the muscle so that it feels solid and stable, but not overly tensed.

Draw your abdomen in and upwards towards your spine

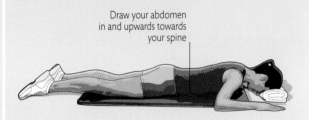

Lie face down on a mat with a rolled-up towel beneath your head, arms beside you, pointing forwards, palms down, your elbows bent at right angles. Draw your abdomen towards your spine in a slow controlled movement, hollowing your middle while keeping your hips and legs relaxed. Aim to contract your transverse abdominis around a third of the way in, so that it feels strong and stable.

CORE TRAINING AND SPORT

Core training is important for sport, as all sports involve core-based movements of one form or another. Because training your core helps your mobility, stability, and strength (»pp.18–19), it will increase the power, efficiency, and consistency of the movements you make, while improving your stability and balance, and reducing your chances of injury.

Strengthening your core helps to stabilize your spine and pelvis. This provides a stronger platform for all of the movements you make, increasing your body's efficiency in transferring power to your limbs. In running, for example, it can help to prevent the forward or backward rotation of your pelvis, which is important because an awkward running gait will cost you speed and increase the chances of injury.

PLANES OF MOVEMENT

All bodily movements occur along three planes – sagittal (vertically forwards and backwards), frontal (vertically side to side), and transverse (horizontally) – with stabilization used to describe a stationary position.

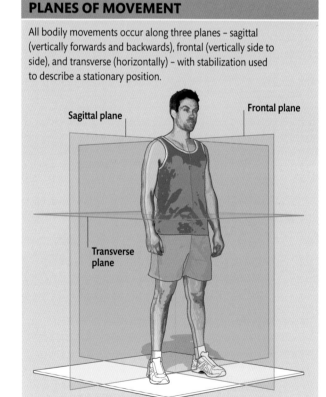

Sagittal plane

Frontal plane

Transverse plane

Meanwhile, in sports that involve throwing movements, such as hammer, shot put, discus, javelin, and fielding in baseball or cricket, the efficient transfer of power to your throwing arm is especially important. Core strength also improves the consistency of your movements because it gives your limbs a stable base from which to work. This is particularly important in sports such as golf and tennis, in which the ability to repeat a movement consistently over the course of a match has a direct bearing on the outcome.

CORE STRENGTH AND BALANCE

Training your core also improves your balance. Most sports – especially team sports that involve running on an uneven pitch – involve movements that are unbalanced. To combat this, sports coaches will use a range of drills and exercises that combine unexpected and varying levels of resistance, with different directions of movement – forwards, backwards, lateral, and vertical. They may also incorporate unstable surfaces in training, using equipment such as stability discs or suspension bodyweight straps (»pp.32–33).

CORE STRENGTH AND INJURY

Ensuring you have a well-developed and balanced core will help to create a strong kinetic chain (»pp.10–11), resulting in all parts of your body working in harmony to improve your performance and achieve your desired goals, while also reducing your chances of muscular imbalances, which can cause both little niggles and more serious injuries.

WHICH CORE EXERCISES ARE BEST FOR MY SPORT?

All sports are different and when designing your own core-training programme you should first analyse the movements that occur in your sport and train your core accordingly. Sports that require a lot of agility, such as football, gymnastics, or snowboarding, will require multi-plane core exercises, whereas sports such as cycling, kayaking, or bobsleigh, will not. However, most athletes will benefit from training the core in all planes of motion to some degree as this helps to stabilize the pelvis and spine, whichis important for all sports. The extent to which you train these planes is dependent on programme design and the amount of time you are able to train. For more information see the sports-specific section (»pp.194–97).

CORE MOVEMENTS AND SPORT

In this book we have divided core-based movements into five main categories: isometric; flexion; extension; side flexion; and rotation. A sixth type, known as complex, represents a movement combining two or more of the others. Movements in most sports could be described as complex, but some examples of the main ones are listed below.

MOVEMENT	CHARACTERISTICS	SPORTS SUCH AS...
Isometric	■ **Plane of movement:** Stabilization ■ **Typical movements:** Holding yourself in a fixed position; resisting an external force, such as a weight, or an opponent ■ **Example exercises:** Plank-based exercises ■ **Exercise benefits:** Strengthens and stabilizes your whole core	■ Boxing ■ Football ■ Wrestling ■ Gymnastics ■ Ice hockey ■ Rowing ■ Rugby league
Flexion	■ **Plane of movement:** Sagittal ■ **Typical movements:** Bending forwards or bending over; moving to sit or stand from a prone position ■ **Example exercises:** Sit-ups and crunches ■ **Exercise benefits:** Strengthens and stabilizes your ribcage and pelvis	■ American football ■ Netball ■ Judo ■ Football ■ Cycling ■ Volleyball
Extension	■ **Plane of movement:** Sagittal ■ **Typical movements:** Bending back to straighten the back from a bent-over position; the arching of the back ■ **Example exercises:** Back extensions; good mornings ■ **Exercise benefits:** Strengthens and stabilizes your back	■ Wrestling ■ High jump ■ Gymnastics ■ Swimming ■ Weightlifting ■ Basketball ■ Pole vaulting
Side Flexion	■ **Plane of movement:** Frontal ■ **Typical movements:** Bending from side to side from the waist; reaching overhead to either side ■ **Example exercises:** Windmills; side bends ■ **Exercise benefits**: Stabilizes your pelvis and improves posture	■ Climbing ■ Skiing ■ Snowboarding ■ Martial arts ■ Squash
Rotation	■ **Plane of movement:** Transverse ■ **Typical movements:** Turning movements; rotating from the waist ■ **Example exercises:** Pulley chops and lifts; super-slow bicycles ■ **Exercise benefits:** Improves your rotational strength and your ability to resist external rotational forces	■ Golf ■ Baseball ■ Softball ■ Shot put ■ Badminton ■ Hammer ■ Canoeing
Complex	■ **Movement plane:** Multi-plane ■ **Typical movements:** Combination actions that include two or more of those core movements detailed above ■ **Example exercises:** Medicine ball chops; Turkish get-ups ■ **Exercise benefits:** Combines the benefits of the movements	■ American football ■ Basketball ■ Tennis ■ Skiing ■ Football ■ Martial arts

CORE TRAINING AND PREGNANCY

Core training during pregnancy can help improve strength, stability, mobility, and balance, all of which may contribute to an expectant mother's overall sense of wellbeing. It will also help relieve back tension and accelerate the recovery of the abdominal muscles after birth.

During pregnancy many changes will happen to your body. Those that affect your spine, shoulder, and pelvic stability will all have an impact on posture and core strength. If this is your first pregnancy you are particularly vulnerable to back pain and injury, as well as experiencing a reduced sense of balance as your bump gets bigger. Hormone imbalances lead to an increase in the elasticity of connective tissues, causing joint instability. Focus on stability and postural strength, and

PREGNANCY AND POST-PREGNANCY CORE-STRENGTH TRAINING

STAGE	WHAT TO EXPECT	THINGS TO WATCH OUT FOR
First trimester (0–12 weeks)	■ Considered to be the most delicate stage of pregnancy, this is when most of the changes to your body start to take place. ■ General changes include an increased metabolic rate; adjustments in hormone levels; fluctuations in mood or emotion; nausea; fatigue or predisposition to clumsiness; decreased blood pressure; pelvic changes; and slight weight gain.	■ An enhanced metabolic rate may cause a significant increase in internal core temperature. In extreme cases, this can lead to foetal hyperthermia (the foetus overheating). ■ Isometric exercises, such as the plank, increase core temperature. You can perform modified versions of them, but relax and breathe evenly throughout.
Second trimester (13–26 weeks)	■ As your uterus becomes heavier to make room for the baby, your abdomen expands and your belly becomes more prominent. ■ This results in a decreased degree of movement and spinal flexibility. Lying flat on your back may become uncomfortable. ■ General changes may include increased energy levels; abdominal discomfort; constipation; heartburn; and back pain.	■ Increased oestrogen, progesterone, and relaxin levels cause ligaments and connective tissues to soften and relax, potentially leading to joint instability. ■ Lumbar spine flexion will be reduced as your bump gets larger, so try to minimize bending from your lower back. ■ Avoid exercises that test lumbar rotation stability and side bends that over-extend the spine.
Third trimester (27–40 weeks)	■ In the late stages of pregnancy the growth of the baby will start to place pressure on the lower abdomen and shift your centre of gravity, altering core balance and postural alignment. Freedom to perform everyday tasks will become restricted due to the size of your bump. ■ General changes that may occur include back pain and shoulder stiffness; fatigue; shortness of breath; sciatica; haemorrhoids; and Braxton Hicks contractions (false labour pain).	■ Exercises that place further pressure on your lower abdomen may lead to incontinence. (Pelvic-floor activation (**»p.56**) may counteract this effect.) ■ Avoid lying on your back for prolonged periods of time. Compression on the vena cava may reduce blood flow to the placenta resulting in supine hypotensive syndrome – symptoms include dizziness and nausea.
Post-pregnancy (6+ weeks after birth)	■ Months of inactivity and overstretched stomach muscles will weaken the abdominals, leaving new mothers prone to back pain or injury, especially if the diastasis recti (**Warning box, top right**) is enlarged. ■ Loss of core strength and balance is inevitable, and stability exercises will play an important part in recovering your pre-pregnancy strength. ■ If you have a Caesarean section, you must seek your doctor's approval before you start exercising again, because Caesarean sections involve cutting through the abdominal muscles.	■ Exercising immediately after birth. Usually you can begin exercising your core six weeks after birth but get clearance from a doctor, midwife, or nurse practitioner first. A diastasis recti check will decide if core training is safe to begin. ■ Avoid spine flexion exercise, such as crunches, if an enlarged diastasis recti (**Warning box, top right**) is present.

be careful not to over-work or over-stretch the joints of your spine and hips. Pilates or a specially-designed core training programme (**»pp.182–85**) can help, but always seek guidance from your doctor or midwife before you begin. The benefits of core-strength training during pregnancy include:

- strengthening the muscles of your pelvic floor, transverse abdominis, hips, and lower back to assist with delivery
- increasing hip and spinal stability
- relieving back pain and tension
- reducing neck and shoulder tension
- accelerating the recovery of core muscles after birth

WARNING!

Diastasis recti is the separation that occurs along the centre line, or linea alba, of the rectus abdominis muscle. A separation of one or two fingers width is normal, but a gap any greater than this is a cause for concern. Performing abdominal (flexion) exercises with an enlarged diastasis recti can cause the rectus abdominis muscle to strengthen and shorten in the separated position. This weakens the abdominal area, causing lower-back pain or injury and a possible risk of hernia. If you are concerned about this condition, seek advice from a doctor.

FOCUS ON	KEY EXERCISE	ADDITIONAL EXERCISES
■ Pelvic-floor education. This is crucial in pregnancy. It is advisable to start activating the pelvic floor as soon as possible. ■ Deep abdominal stability to strengthen your back and improve your balance. ■ Exercises such as the dart (**»p.65**) to promote shoulder stability and alignment.	■ **Active pelvic floor** (**»p.56**) Improves core and hip stability throughout pregnancy. Also helps to maintain urinary and bowel continence in the later stages of pregnancy, and aids in the preparation for delivery. 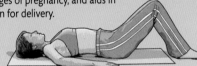	■ **Knee fold** (**»p.60**) ■ **Dart** (**»p.65**) ■ **Star** (**»p.68**)
■ Core stability, especially of your hips and lumbar spine. Pillow squeezes (**»p.58**) and bridges (**»p.98**) are particularly good exercises for this. ■ Pelvic-floor activation to help support the position of the baby.	■ **Bridge** (**»p.98**) Activates and strengthens the muscles of your lower back and hips, helping to stabilize your pelvis, improving pregnancy postures, and even helping reduce back pain.	■ **Child's pose** (**»p.52**) ■ **Pillow squeeze** (**»p.58**) ■ **Heel slide** (**»p.59**)
■ Core-training exercises that help prepare for the delivery. ■ Strengthening your core and hip stability. Practise the four-point kneeling position, with your hands placed on the floor in front of you. This will encourage your baby into the correct position. Supermans (**»p.70**) will also help with this.	■ **Superman** (**»p.70**) Improves your core balance, strengthens your pelvic floor connection and back muscles, works to stabilize your hips, and helps your baby into the correct position.	■ **Shoulder rotation** (**»p.47**) ■ **Oyster** (**»p.66**) ■ **Cat stretch** (**»p.168**)
■ Strengthening your pelvic floor, abdominal muscles, and improving your posture. ■ Stability exercises, as you will still have increased levels of relaxin for months after the birth. ■ Activation and foundation level exercises, before gradually building up core strength over a period of about nine months.	■ **Prone abdominal hollowing** (**»p.64**) Builds the strength of the deep abdominal muscles. Helps in the support of the lower back and can be a positive influence on the repair of the diastasis recti (**Warning box, top right**). 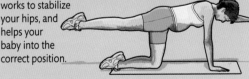	■ **Toe tap** (**»p.62**) ■ **Dorsal raise** (**»p.76**) ■ **Plank** (**»pp.102–03**)

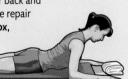

ASSESSING YOUR CORE

Regardless of your core-training goals, you will achieve much more if you think carefully and strategically about achieving a balanced training programme from the start.

The first step of your training should be to perform an assessment of your core. This will help you to identify any areas which require improvement, so you can target weaknesses and structure your training accordingly.

CORE STRENGTH ASSESSMENT

The following exercises challenge your core in a variety of ways, and can be used as a basic assessment to measure your core strength. Ask a partner to observe you and assess your form throughout, identifying any movements you're unable to carry out with good technique. To resolve any areas of weakness, you should practise the recommended exercises, repeating the test regularly to gauge your improvements.

Toe tap (»pp.62–63)
■ You should be able to: ▶ perform the exercise without extension in your lower back.
■ If you can't, you should focus on:
▶ strengthening your abs and back to help stabilize your lumbar spine with exercises such as knee folds (»pp.60–61), darts (»p.65), and supermans (»pp.70–71).

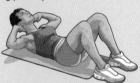

Abdominal crunch (»pp.72–73)
■ You should be able to: ▶ perform the exercise without flattening your back or tucking your hips.
■ If you can't, you should focus on:
▶ achieving correct hip placement and lumbar stability with exercises such as heel slides (»p.59), reverse curls (»p.75), and stars (»p.68).

Side-lying leg lift (»pp.84–85)
■ You should be able to: ▶ keep your spine stationary and aligned.
■ If you can't, you should focus on: ▶ strengthening your lumbar spine and glutes against side flexion and rotational forces with exercises such as supermans (»pp.70–71), side bends (»p.81), and heel reaches (»p.82).

Bridge with knee lift (»p.99)
■ You should be able to: ▶ keep your spine aligned without rotating or dropping your hips.
■ If you can't, you should focus on:
▶ strengthening your glutes, lower back, and deep abdominals with exercises such as oysters (»p.66), prone leg lifts (»p.67), and planks (»pp.102–03).

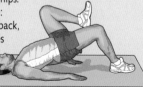

Plank (»pp.102–03)
■ You should be able to: ▶ perform the exercise without sagging through your spine, dropping your hips, or rotating your lower back.
■ If you can't, you should focus on: ▶ strengthening your glutes, lumbar spine, and deep abdominals with exercises such as darts (»p.65), supermans (»pp.70–71), and bridges (»pp.98–99).

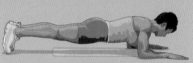

Hip roll (»pp.88–89)
■ You should be able to: ▶ perform the exercise without rotating your upper body.
■ If you can't, you should focus on:
▶ stabilizing your lumbar spine and strengthening your abs with supermans (»pp.70–71), oblique reaches (»pp.86–87), and super-slow bicycles (»p.95).

Leg circle (»p.74)
■ You should be able to: ▶ keep your spine and hips aligned while moving your leg.
■ If you can't you should focus on: ▶ strengthening your deep abdominals, internal obliques, and deep glutes with exercises such as oysters (»p.66), stars (»p.68), and horizontal balances (»p.97).

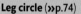

Swim (»p.94)
■ You should be able to: ▶ maintain your spine and hip alignment without rotating your body, while moving your arms and legs.
■ If you can't, you should focus on: ▶ stabilizing and strengthening the muscles of your lower back, deep abdominals, and glutes with exercises such as stars (»p.68), supermans (»pp.70–71), and planks (»pp.102–03).

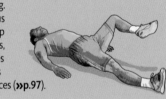

DEVELOPING YOUR CORE

The primary purpose of the core is to provide mobility, stability, strength, and balance to the mid-section of your body. This creates a more stable and powerful platform for movement throughout the rest of your body.

Developing core strength is a gradual process. All of the exercises in this book are designed to test your strength at the same time as you develop it, and, as your training progresses, you will notice an improvement in your performance. Be patient in your approach to training, in order to build a solid base of core strength before you attempt any more advanced exercises.

ACTIVATING YOUR CORE

The first stage of your core training should involve learning how to engage your key core muscles and achieve a neutral pelvic position (**»p.25**). You should then focus on "activating" your core using the exercises in the Activation section of this book (**»pp.56–71**). At first you should work on the core in isolation, then start to incorporate it into more challenging movements. At this stage, you should keep your training simple – do not be tempted to push yourself too far, too quickly.

FOUNDATION-LEVEL CORE TRAINING

Once you have learned to activate your core, you can progress to a selection of simple bodyweight exercises, in which movement is limited to a single plane of motion such as side to side, or forwards and backwards. These are the exercises most people traditionally think of in relation to core training and include sit-ups, back extensions, and planks. Remember, even as you reach an intermediate level of training, the simplest programme is usually the best.

INTERMEDIATE AND ADVANCED CORE TRAINING

When you have achieved a basic level of core stability and strength, you can move to more complex single and multi-plane exercises using instability equipment, such as exercise balls, and weights to increase the difficulty of your programme. These exercises should be used to test your core to its maximum ability and include medicine ball slams, kettlebell swings, and suspended bodyweight crunches.

TESTING YOUR CORE

Depending on which core muscles you want to train, you first have to know which movements to perform regularly and which muscles are active during these movements. This knowledge and understanding will help you to design a balanced programme that incorporates all core muscles and movement types to maintain a strong and balanced core.

DEFINITION OF DIFFICULTY LEVELS

The exercises in this book have been awarded a difficulty level of 1-10, according to the following definitions. You should aim to progress through Levels 1-4 (Activation and Foundation) before you move on to Level 5-10 (Intermediate and Advanced) as it is crucial to have a good general level of core strength before you attempt complex, multi-joint movements.

Activation	
Level 1	Basic-level exercises that "wake up" the muscles of the core
Foundation	
Level 2	Exercises using bodyweight only
Level 3	Bodyweight exercises with limb movement, and/or varied speed of movement
Level 4	Isometric exercises
Intermediate	
Level 5	Loaded exercises and isometric exercises with limb movements
Level 6	Power exercises and suspended bodyweight exercises
Level 7	Isometric and complex exercises requiring good core strength
Advanced	
Level 8	Exercises involving external weight and full body extension
Level 9	Cable-based exercises with added instability
Level 10	Challenging exercises utilizing all movement types. (These require excellent core and full body strength and should not be attempted by novices.)

EQUIPMENT FOR CORE TRAINING

There are numerous pieces of equipment that you can use to increase the difficulty of exercises by adding weight or instability. However, it is important for you to master each of the basic movements first to ensure you are using the correct core muscles, before incorporating some weighted and unstable progressions into your core-training regimen.

PROGRESSING EXERCISES WITH WEIGHT

You can make an exercise more challenging by adding weight to the movement with equipment such as a medicine ball, kettlebell, or dumbbell. Extra weight increases the force the active or "working" muscles are required to produce – in other words, the heavier the weight the harder the exercise. However, you should never increase weight at the expense of your form or technique, as this will only increase your chances of sustaining an injury. You should only add weight once you can first perform the basic bodyweight exercise with good form for several reps and sets. When adding weight, you should aim to increase the load in increments of around 1–2kg (2.2–4.4lb) at a time to allow your body to adapt. Jumping from a 2kg (4.4lb) kettlebell to one weighing 10kg (22lb), for example, will stress your muscles and joints beyond their comfortable working ability.

PROGRESSING EXERCISES WITH INSTABILITY

In most cases you will first perform the basic version of an exercise on the floor or a stable surface, such as a weight bench. Once you have mastered this basic movement, however, you can make it harder by gradually increasing the level of instability. This may involve adjusting your body position to remove the support of your arms or legs, or reducing the stability of the surface bearing your weight by using a piece of gym equipment such as a stability disc or exercise ball. The unstable surface makes your core work harder or in a slightly different way to keep your body balanced. The table on the right ranks common pieces of equipment in increasing instability to help you decide what to use. It is important to note that the most effective way of progressing exercise is sometimes achieved by increasing instability, rather than by adding weight.

"FUNCTIONAL" CORE TRAINING

Instability training is sometimes referred to as "functional training". The basic premise of functional training is that performing an exercise on a less stable base not only requires more work to be done by the primary working muscles you are targeting, but it also brings into play a number of other muscles to help to control and to stabilize the movement. These muscles are known as neutralizers and fixators (or stabilizers), and include both the core muscles and the smaller muscles of the limbs.

It is important to remember that these smaller, stabilizing muscle groups tire more quickly than the primary working muscles, meaning that less force can be applied to them, and less work completed by them. Instability training is therefore not appropriate for strengthening a single muscle group to its maximum, as this will lead to under-performance and reduced gains in strength. Instead, it is designed to train the body as a whole, strengthening and harmonizing the kinetic chain (**»pp.10–11**) to maximize performance and reduce the risk of injury. Your core muscles help to stabilize your spine, ensuring the efficient transfer of strength and stability to your limbs during movements. It is this that will give you the combination of strength, stability, and mobility required to perform some of the more challenging core exercises in this book, such as hanging toe tucks (**»p.150**), Turkish get-ups (**»pp.156–57**), and wall walks (**»pp.164–65**).

CORE TRAINING AND INSTABILITY

When adding instability to make an exercise harder (as in many of the progressions included in this book), it is useful to think in relative terms – for example, whether one piece of equipment offers more or less instability and freedom of movement than another. The following list ranks a number of options in order of increasing instability (the most stable at the top) to help you to assess and choose the appropriate exercise progression.

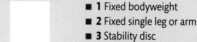

- **1** Fixed bodyweight
- **2** Fixed single leg or arm
- **3** Stability disc
- **4** Wobble board
- **5** Half-exercise ball
- **6** Exercise ball
- **7** Suspended bodyweight straps

EQUIPMENT FOR EFFECTIVE CORE TRAINING

EQUIPMENT THAT ADDS INSTABILITY

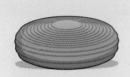

Stability disc
■ A cushion-sized inflatable disc that can be inflated/deflated to the required thickness to provide a simple unstable platform for basic instability exercises.

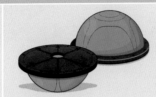

Half-exercise ball
■ This combines half of a small inflatable ball with a hard platform. You can use the device as a support on both sides, but using it ball side down creates greater instabilty.

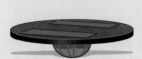

Wobble board
■ A platform designed to tilt in any direction. It offers less stability than a half-exercise ball, because the "ball" on the underside is smaller and made of a hard material.

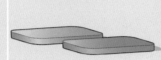

Slide board
■ Slide boards are usually used in pairs to add an element of lateral instability, because they can slip along the floor in all directions when weight is placed on them.

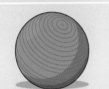

Exercise ball
■ A large inflatable ball that rolls in all directions, and therefore offers very little stability. Choose one with a diameter roughly the same as the length of your arm.

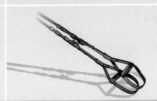

Bodyweight suspension strap
■ Fixed to a stable rack or bar, these straps suspend your arms or legs in the air, removing their support to increase the instability of an exercise.

EQUIPMENT THAT ADDS WEIGHT

Kettlebell
■ A cannonball-shaped weight with a different centre of gravity to a dumbbell. It can be held in one or both hands, and used for dynamic strength exercises.

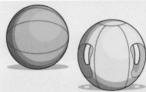

Medicine ball
■ A football-sized weighted ball that may come with or without handles. It is primarily used for exercises that build dynamic strength and power.

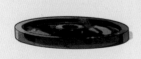
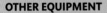

Weight disc
■ These are usually added in pairs to barbells and dumbbells, but can also be used as a hand-held weight, or as a weighted object to be pushed along the ground.

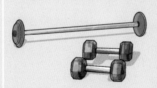

Barbell/Dumbbell
■ The most common form of weights for strength training: barbells are designed to be lifted with both hands, and dumbbells with one.

OTHER EQUIPMENT

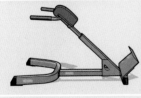

Roman chair
■ A piece of equipment that is used to hold the feet and legs in position in order to isolate and work the muscles of the lower back and glutes.

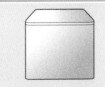

Box
■ A simple stable platform of various sizes. It can be used to add height to dynamic exercises, or raise supporting limbs to increase instability.

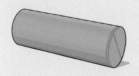

Foam roller
■ A cylinder of dense foam, the roller can be used to perform self-massage on tight muscles, and also as an unstable base that moves backwards and forwards.

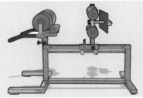

GHD
■ Similar to the Roman chair, the GHD (glute-hamstring developer) fixes your limbs in place to target the muscles of your lower back, glutes, and hamstrings.

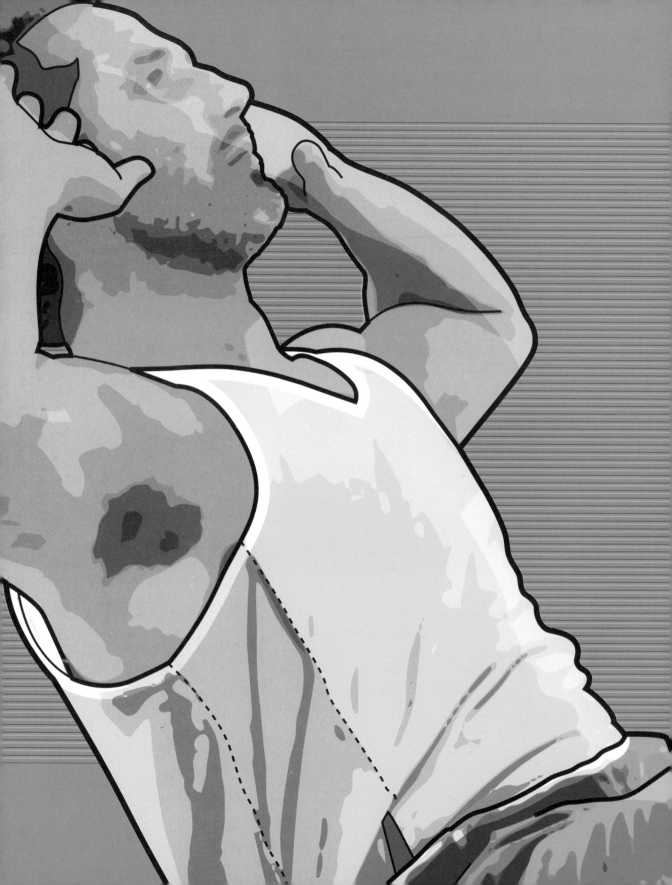

CORE-TRAINING EXERCISES

2

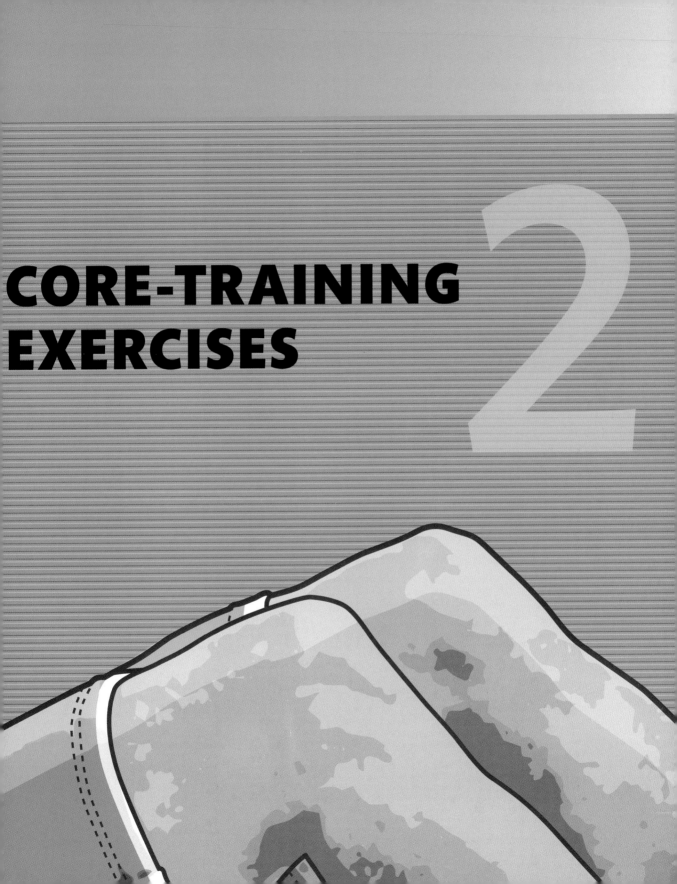

VISUAL EXERCISE DIRECTORY

ACTIVATION EXERCISES

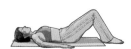

Active Pelvic Floor
»pp.56–57

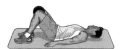

Pillow Squeeze
»p.58

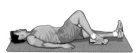

Heel Slide
»p.59

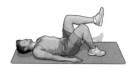

Knee Fold
»pp.60–61

FOUNDATION EXERCISES

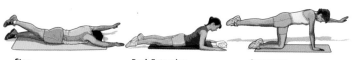

Star
»p.68

Back Extension
»p.69

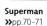

Superman
»pp.70–71

Abdominal Crunch
»pp.72–73

Leg Circle
»p.74

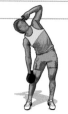

Side Bend
»p.81

Heel Reach
»p.82

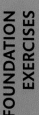

Roman Chair Side Bend
»p.83

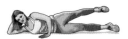

Side-lying Leg Lift
»pp.84–85

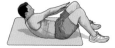

Oblique Reach
»pp.86–87

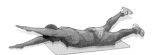

Swim
»p.94

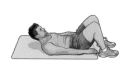

Super-slow Bicycle
»p.95

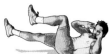

Sprinter Sit-up
»p.96

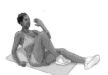

Horizontal Balance
»p.97

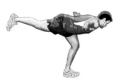

Bridge
»pp.98–99

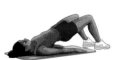

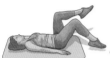

Toe Tap
>>pp.62–63

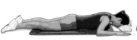

Prone Abdominal Hollowing >>p.64

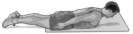

Dart
>>p.65

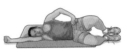

Oyster
>>p.66

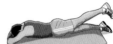

Prone Leg Lift
>>p.67

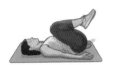

Reverse Curl
>>p.75

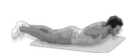

Dorsal Raise
>>pp.76–77

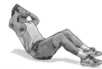

Sit-up
>>p.78

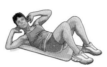

Oblique Crunch
>>p.79

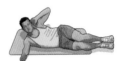

Side-lying Lateral Crunch
>>p.80

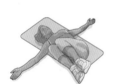

Hip Roll
>>pp.88–89

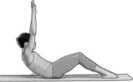

Roll-back
>>p.90

Roll-up
>>p.91

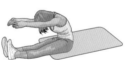

V Leg-raise
>>p.92

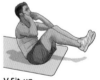

V Sit-up
>>p.93

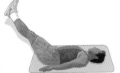

Double-leg Lower and Lift >>pp.100–01

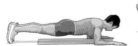

Plank
>>pp.102–03

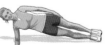

Side Plank
>>pp.104–05

Single-leg Extension and Stretch >>p.106

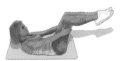

Double-leg Extension and Stretch >>p.107

INTERMEDIATE EXERCISES

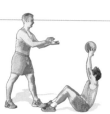

Partner Ball Swap
>>pp.108–09

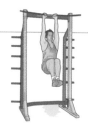

**Hanging
Knee-up** >>pp.110–11

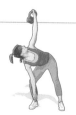

Windmill
>>pp.110–11

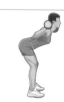

Good Morning
>>pp.112–13

**Roman Chair Back
Extension** >>pp.112–13

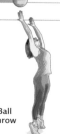

**Medicine Ball
Reverse Throw**
>>p.121

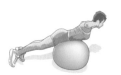

**Exercise Ball Back
Extension** >>p.122

Medicine Ball Bridge
>>p.123

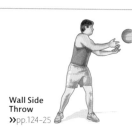

**Wall Side
Throw**
>>pp.124–25

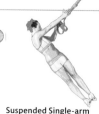

**Suspended Single-arm
Core Rotation** >>p.126

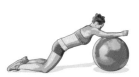

**Exercise Ball
Roll-out** >>pp.132–33

Suspended Crunch
>>p.134

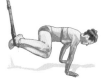

**Suspended Oblique
Crunch** >>p.135

Medicine Ball Chop
>>p.136

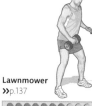

Lawnmower
>>p.137

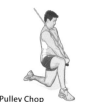

Pulley Chop
>>pp.144–45

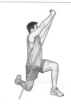

Pulley Lift
>>pp.146–47

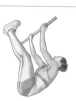

**Single-leg, Single-arm
Cable Press** >>pp.148–49

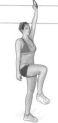

**Hanging Toe
Tuck** >>p.150

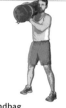

**Sandbag
Shouldering** >>p.151

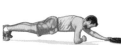

Plank Plate Push
>>pp.152–53

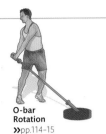

O-bar Rotation
≫pp.114–15

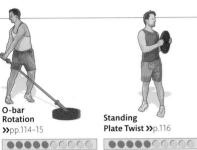

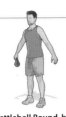

Standing Plate Twist ≫p.116

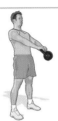

Kettlebell Round-body Swing ≫p.117

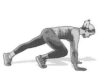

Mountain Climber
≫p.118

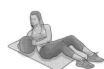

Russian Twist
≫p.119

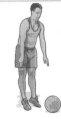

Medicine Ball Slam
≫p.120

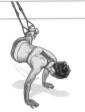

Suspended Pendulum
≫p.127

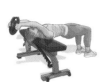

Long-arm Bridge Pull-over ≫p.128

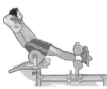

Kettlebell Swing
≫p.129

Exercise Ball Knee Tuck ≫p.130

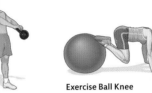

Core Board Rotation ≫p.131

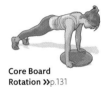

ADVANCED EXERCISES

GHD Sit-up
≫p.138

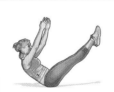

Pike
≫p.139

Stick Crunch
≫pp.140–41

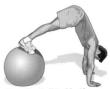

Exercise Ball Jackknife
≫p.142

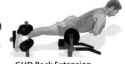

GHD Back Extension
≫p.143

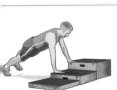

Stepped Plank Walk
≫pp.154–55

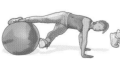

Turkish Get-up with Kettlebell
≫pp.156–57

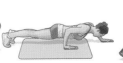

Exercise Ball Hip Rotation Kick
≫pp.158–59

Slide Board Wiper
≫pp.160–61

Raised Pike Dumbbell Hand-walk ≫pp.162–63

Wall Walk
≫pp.164–65

CORE MOVEMENT DIRECTORY

As you begin to train your core muscles using the exercises in this section, it is important to think of each in terms of their core movement, as well as their level difficulty. This is a key part of understanding how your core muscles work together, and to achieving the best results in your training. Using a balanced combination of movements will help you to gain excellent overall strength, stability, and mobility, while reducing the likelihood of muscular imbalance and injury.

The Core Exercise Matrix on the next few pages is designed to offer quick, user-friendly reference to help you locate the exercises in the book according to their core movement, along with details of the number of progressions they have.

The six core movements are ordered in the same way that they appear in the key at the start of the book (»p.9): Isometric; Flexion; Extension; Side Flexion; Rotation; and Complex; the individual exercises are then ordered presented according to their level of difficulty and page order. It is important to note that while Isometric exercises come first and there are more of them than for the other movements, this does not mean that they are more important. Balance is the key when you are training your core and you should always endeavour to combine as many core movements as you can.

USING THE MATRIX

The chart on the following pages groups exercises in the main section of this chapter (»pp.56–165) according to their Target Movement, ranking them in order of Difficulty Level, and listing the number of progressions for each. You can use this information in conjunction with the Design Your Own programmes (»pp.186–89) if you are looking for exercises of a specific movement and level, the Sports-Specific chapter (»pp.192–215) if you are intending to train specific core movements for your chosen sport, or simply as a general reference to help with your training. It is important to remember that you should always train using a selection of exercises from a balanced range of core movements.

CORE EXERCISE MATRIX

ISOMETRIC EXERCISES

EXERCISE	LEVEL	PROGRESSIONS	PAGE
Active Pelvic Floor	1	2	56–57
Pillow Squeeze	1	2	58
Heel Slide	1	–	59
Knee Fold	1	1	60–61
Toe Tap	1	4	62–63
Prone Abdominal Hollowing	1	–	64
Oyster	1	–	66
Prone Leg Lift	1	–	67
Star	1	–	68
Superman	1	4	70–71

Leg Circle	2	1	74	Core Board Rotation	7	1	131
Side-lying Leg Lift	2	1	84–85	Single-leg, Single-arm Cable Press	9	–	148–49
Swim	3	–	94	Plank Plate Push	10	–	152–53
Horizontal Balance	4	1	97	Stepped Plank Walk	10	–	154–55
Bridge	4	5	98–99				
Double-leg Lower and Lift	4	3	100–01				

FLEXION EXERCISES

EXERCISE	LEVEL	PROGRESSIONS	PAGE

Plank	4	6	102–03	Abdominal Crunch	2	6	72–73
Side Plank	4	3	104–05	Reverse Curl	2	2	75
Kettlebell Round-body Swing	5	–	117	Sit-up	2	1	78
Moutain Climber	5	–	118	Roll-back	2	–	90
Long-arm Bridge Pull-over	7	1	128	Roll-up	3	–	91
Kettlebell Swing	7	–	129	V Leg-raise	3	–	92
Exercise Ball Knee Tuck	7	–	130	V Leg Sit-up	3	–	93

Exercise	Level	Progressions	Page
Sprinter Sit-up	3	–	96
Single–leg Extension and Stretch	4	–	106
Double–leg Extension and Stretch	4	1	107
Partner Ball Swap	5	1	108–09
Hanging Knee-up	5	1	110–11
Medicine Ball Slam	6	–	120
GHD Sit-up	8	–	138
Pike	8	–	139
Stick Crunch	8	–	140–41
Exercise Ball Jack-knife	8	–	142
Hanging Toe Tuck	10	–	150

EXTENSION EXERCISES

EXERCISE	LEVEL	PROGRESSIONS	PAGE
Dart	1	1	65
Back Extension	1	–	69
Dorsal Raise	2	2	76–77
Good Morning	5	–	112–13
Roman Chair Back Extension	5	–	112–13
Medicine Ball Reverse Throw	6	–	121
Exercise Ball Back Extension	6	–	122
GHD Back Extension	8	–	143

SIDE-FLEXION EXERCISES

EXERCISE	LEVEL	PROGRESSIONS	PAGE
Side–lying Lateral Crunch	2	–	80
Side Bend	2	–	81
Heel Reach	2	–	82
Roman Chair Side Bend	2	–	83
Windmill	5	–	110–11

ROTATION EXERCISES

EXERCISE	LEVEL	PROGRESSIONS	PAGE
Oblique Crunch	2	1	79
Oblique Reach	2	4	86–87
Hip Roll	2	3	88–89
Super-slow Bicycle	3	–	95
O-bar Rotation	5	–	114–15
Standing Plate Twist	5	–	116
Russian Twist	6	–	119
Medicine Ball Bridge	6	–	123
Wall Side Throw	6	2	124–25
Suspended Single-arm Core Rotation	6	–	126
Pulley Chop	9	3	144–45
Pulley Lift	9	3	146–47

COMPLEX EXERCISES

EXERCISE	LEVEL	PROGRESSIONS	PAGE
Suspended Pendulum	7	–	127
Exercise Ball Roll-out	7	1	132–33
Suspended Crunch	7	1	134
Suspended Oblique Crunch	7	–	135
Medicine Ball Chop	7	–	136
Lawnmower	7	–	137
Sandbag Shouldering	10	–	151
Turkish Get-up with Kettlebell	10	–	156–57
Exercise Ball Hip Rotation Kick	10	2	158–59
Slide Board Wiper	10	–	160–61
Raised Pike Dumbbell Hand-walk	10	3	162–63
Wall Walk	10	–	164–65

MOBILIZATION

Mobility stretches are a key part of any exercise routine, helping you to get the best results and reducing your risk of injury. They lengthen and loosen your muscles, increasing your range of movement and flexibility, and reducing stiffness and pressure on your discs, ligaments, and facet joints. When performing the movements, relax your body, and breathe deeply and rhythmically.

THORACIC ROLLER

In this exercise, the foam roller acts as a hinge to help improve the range of motion in your middle and upper back. It is a good movement to mobilize the muscles of your neck and back.

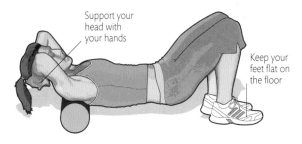

Support your head with your hands

Keep your feet flat on the floor

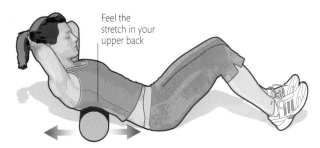

Feel the stretch in your upper back

1 Sit with your heels planted on the floor and the roller beneath the middle of your back. Lie back onto the roller so that it is just below your shoulder blades. Clasp your hands together and lightly cradle your head.

2 With your chin tucked in, slide up and down the roller, from your neck down to the level of your lowest ribs, but do not go too low into your lumbar spine. Repeat the exercise for at least 30 seconds.

LAT ROLLER

This exercise helps to loosen up the large muscles of your middle and upper back, reducing tightness, tension, and muscular pain.

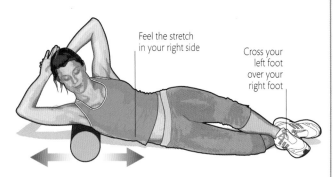

Feel the stretch in your right side

Cross your left foot over your right foot

Lie on your right side with the roller positioned beneath your armpit, and place your hands behind your head for stability. Use your back muscles to roll down from your armpit to the base of your shoulder blade. Roll back up and repeat for at least 30 seconds, then switch sides.

GLUTE/PIRIFORMIS ROLLER

This exercise loosens up the gluteals at the outside of your buttocks and the piriformis towards the middle of them.

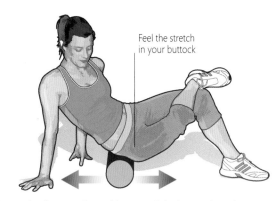

Feel the stretch in your buttock

Sit on the foam roller with your right buttock and cross your right leg over your left leg. Rolling backwards and forwards, work on the outside of your buttock before shifting your weight to the middle of your buttock. Repeat for at least 30 seconds before switching sides.

LUMBAR ROLLER

In this exercise, the foam roller works the muscles of your lumbar spine, helping to mobilize your lower back. A strong lower back is essential for all sports, from running to weightlifting, and is important for anyone who spends a lot of time working at a desk.

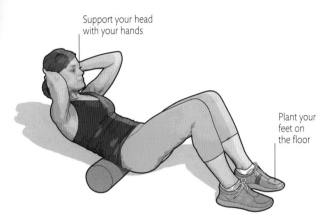

Support your head with your hands

Plant your feet on the floor

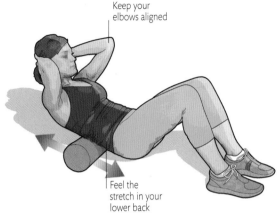

Keep your elbows aligned

Feel the stretch in your lower back

1 Sit with your heels planted on the floor and the roller positioned beneath your lower back. Place your hands on either side of your head and cradle it lightly, without putting any strain on your neck.

2 Keeping your head stable, slowly and carefully slide up and down on the roller, from the bottom of your ribcage to the top of your pelvis. Repeat for at least 30 seconds.

TFL/ITB ROLLER

This exercise loosens your iliotibial band (ITB), the band of muscular tissue on the outside of your upper leg, and helps general mobility in your glutes and hip muscles. It also loosens your tensor fasciae lata (TFL), a muscle in the thigh that is utilized in sports from hurdling to horse riding.

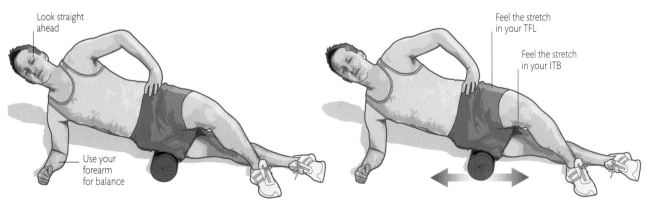

Look straight ahead

Use your forearm for balance

Feel the stretch in your TFL

Feel the stretch in your ITB

1 Lie on your right side with the roller positioned beneath the outside of your thigh, just below your hip. Propping yourself up on your right forearm, with your left hand on your hip, cross your left leg over the right, placing your left foot flat on the floor for support.

2 Using your right forearm, gently push your body over the roller so that the outside of your right thigh slides up and down the roller, as far as your knee. Slide back the opposite way to your hip. Repeat for at least 30 seconds, then swap sides.

NECK ROTATION

This very simple movement can help ease neck aches. After a little practice, you should be able to rotate your neck through at least 70 degrees to each side without feeling "pulls" or hearing cracking sounds.

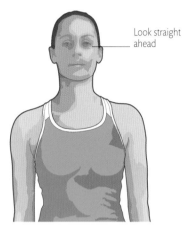

Look straight ahead

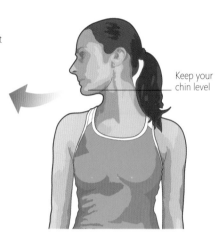

Keep your chin level

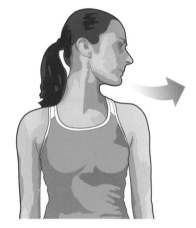

1 Look straight ahead, keeping your spine in a neutral position. Keep the upper body relaxed and your arms loose by your sides.

2 Move your head slowly towards your right shoulder, without straining. Turn it as far as is comfortable and hold for a few seconds.

3 Move your head back through the starting position towards your left shoulder, without straining. Return to the start position.

NECK EXTENSION AND FLEXION

This simple dynamic stretch, which can be carried out standing or seated, will help prevent general neck stiffness and is useful for sports in which head position and movement are important.

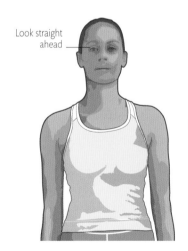

Look straight ahead

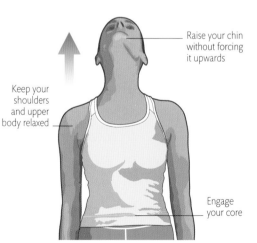

Raise your chin without forcing it upwards

Keep your shoulders and upper body relaxed

Engage your core

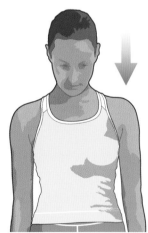

1 Stand upright with your arms by your sides in a relaxed posture. Look straight ahead and keep your spine in a neutral position.

2 Extend your neck as far as is comfortable by slowly raising your chin so you are looking directly upwards. Hold for a few seconds.

3 Flex your neck by letting your head drop forwards without straining. Hold for a few seconds and return to the start position.

NECK SIDE FLEXION

This is a useful mobility stretch for the muscles of your shoulders and neck, helping to ease tightness and tension.

It is also good for mobilizing your spine, and so for improving your posture.

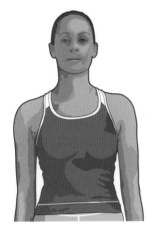
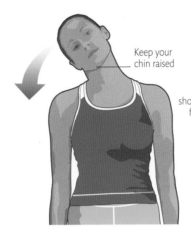
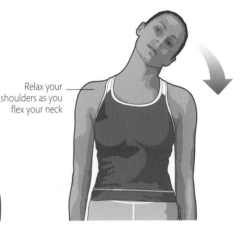

Keep your chin raised

Relax your shoulders as you flex your neck

1 Stand upright, holding your body in a relaxed posture, with your shoulders loose and your eyes looking straight ahead.

2 Tilt your head so that your right ear moves towards your right shoulder as far as is comfortable. Hold for a few seconds.

3 Flex your neck in the opposite direction as far as you can go. Hold for a few seconds and return to the start position.

SHOULDER ROTATION

This exercise provides an excellent way of freeing up the muscles and ligaments around your shoulder joints, and

of warming your trapezius muscles. This is particularly important before beginning a resistance training session.

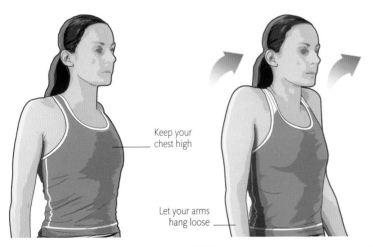
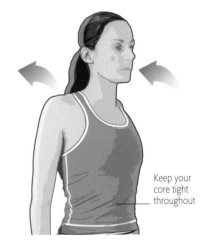

Keep your chest high

Let your arms hang loose

Keep your core tight throughout

1 Let your arms hang loose by your sides and relax your shoulders. Keep your head level and your spine in a neutral position.

2 Rotate your shoulders forwards and up, raising them slowly towards your ears.

3 Hold the position for a few seconds, then reverse the movement backwards.

TORSO ROTATION

This exercise is a useful rotational dynamic stretch for mobilizing your core muscles. Be sure that you keep your hips stationary throughout.

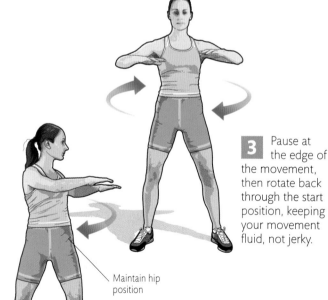

Keep your shoulders relaxed

1 Stand with your feet shoulder-width apart and your elbows raised to each side.

Rotate from the hip

2 Keeping your hips straight and aligned, rotate your upper body with a smooth motion to your right.

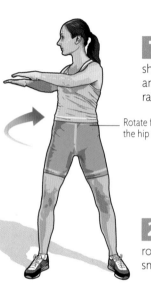

3 Pause at the edge of the movement, then rotate back through the start position, keeping your movement fluid, not jerky.

Maintain hip position

4 Continue the movement to your left side, keeping your hips and your elbows raised to each side. Pause at the edge of the movement, then rotate to the start position.

TORSO SIDE FLEXION

This is a great mobilizing stretch for the muscles of your obliques and upper back. To get the full benefit of the movement, elongate both sides of your torso as you reach up, and avoid leaning forwards.

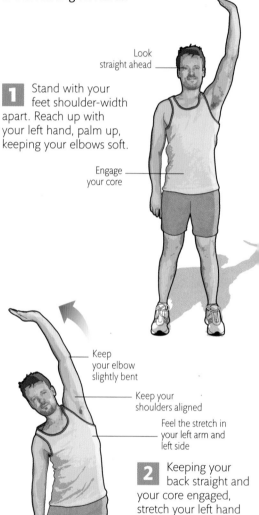

Look straight ahead

1 Stand with your feet shoulder-width apart. Reach up with your left hand, palm up, keeping your elbows soft.

Engage your core

Keep your elbow slightly bent

Keep your shoulders aligned

Feel the stretch in your left arm and left side

2 Keeping your back straight and your core engaged, stretch your left hand up and over your head, reaching down towards your right foot with your right hand. Hold briefly, then release to return to the start position. Repeat as required, before switching arms.

LYING TRUNK ROTATION

This exercise helps to improve the rotational mobility of your upper-back muscles and your thoracic spine, while also stretching the muscles of your chest.

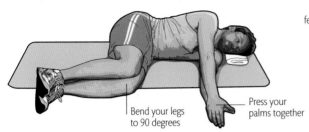

Bend your legs to 90 degrees

Press your palms together

1 Lie on your left side with your hips, knees, and feet stacked one above the other, and your hips and knees bent at right angles. Extend your arms straight in front of you, pressing your palms together.

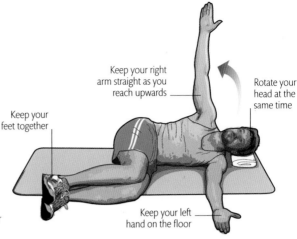

Keep your right arm straight as you reach upwards

Rotate your head at the same time

Keep your feet together

Keep your left hand on the floor

2 Keeping your knees and feet together and your hips stacked, breathe in, brace your abdomen, and reach upwards and back with your right hand, while keeping your left arm straight and resting on the floor.

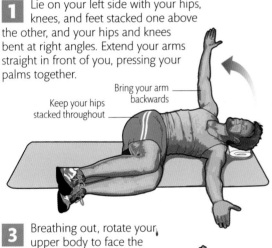

Bring your arm backwards

Keep your hips stacked throughout

3 Breathing out, rotate your upper body to face the ceiling, keeping your hips stacked and your right arm extended.

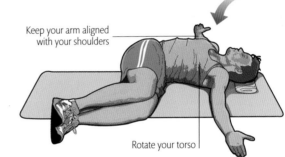

Keep your arm aligned with your shoulders

Rotate your torso

4 Continue the movement until you are as far back as possible, with your chest facing upwards and your hips still stacked. Hold the movement briefly, keeping your shoulders stable and level. Breathe in.

Keep your core engaged

5 Breathing out, reach back towards the ceiling with your right arm, while rotating your torso back towards the start position slowly and under control.

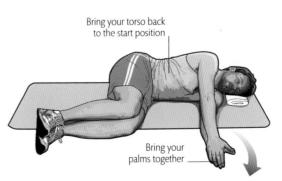

Bring your torso back to the start position

Bring your palms together

6 Continue the movement towards the start position and touch the palms of your hands together. Repeat the movement as required, then switch sides.

LYING WAIST TWIST

This exercise increases the mobility of the joints and muscles in your lower and upper back. Perform the same number of repetitions on both sides of your body.

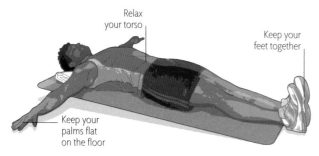

Relax your torso

Keep your feet together

Keep your palms flat on the floor

1 Placing a folded towel under your head for extra support, lie on your back with your body relaxed and your arms loose but extended at a 90-degree angle from your upper body. Keep your legs and feet together.

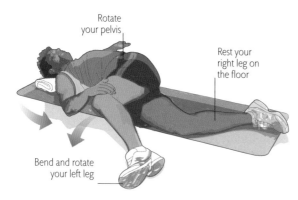

Rotate your pelvis

Rest your right leg on the floor

Bend and rotate your left leg

2 Keeping your upper body flat against the mat, bend your left leg at the knee and bring it across your body, using your right hand to increase the stretch, and allowing your right leg to turn and bend in the same direction.

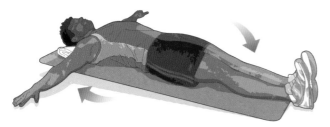

3 Hold the stretch for a few seconds, return to the start position, and switch sides.

CAT AND CAMEL

A great muscle-releasing exercise, this stretch helps to lubricate your spine and get your spinal discs moving. It is one of the best exercises you can do as part of a general warm-up.

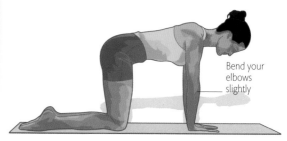

Bend your elbows slightly

1 Kneel on all fours with your hands flat on the floor and in line with your shoulders, your fingers pointing forwards, and your knees below your hips.

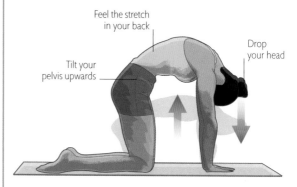

Feel the stretch in your back

Drop your head

Tilt your pelvis upwards

2 Round your back upwards and pull in your stomach, letting your head drop down as you do so. Hold the stretch for a few seconds at the top of the movement.

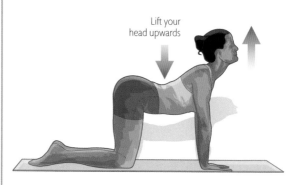

Lift your head upwards

3 In one fluid movement, raise your buttocks and curve your spine downwards while lifting your head so that you are looking straight ahead. Hold the stretch for a few seconds, then return to the start position.

THREADING THE NEEDLE

This dynamic stretch is good for mobilizing the spine and improving your spinal flexibility while warming up the muscles of your shoulders and lower back.

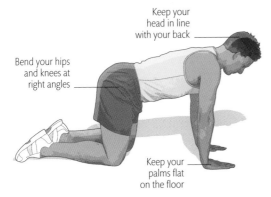

Keep your head in line with your back

Bend your hips and knees at right angles

Keep your palms flat on the floor

1 Kneel on all fours with your back flat and your neck in a relaxed position. Position your arms directly under your shoulders, and bend your hips and knees at right angles, keeping your feet together.

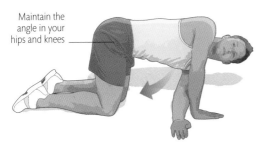

Maintain the angle in your hips and knees

2 Supporting your weight with your right hand, reach under and across your chest with your left hand, turning your head to look to the right.

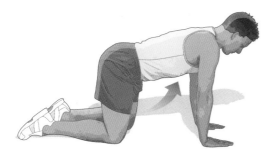

3 Hold the stretch for a few seconds then reverse the movement to the start position. Repeat as required and switch sides.

HIP FLEXOR STRETCH

This stretch is an excellent movement for your hip flexors, which may be particularly tight if you spend a lot of time sitting down. Good hip mobility is vital for balance and posture.

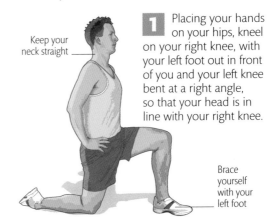

Keep your neck straight

1 Placing your hands on your hips, kneel on your right knee, with your left foot out in front of you and your left knee bent at a right angle, so that your head is in line with your right knee.

Brace yourself with your left foot

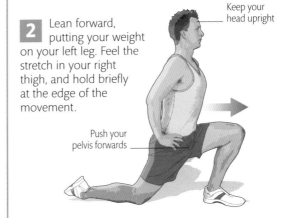

Keep your head upright

2 Lean forward, putting your weight on your left leg. Feel the stretch in your right thigh, and hold briefly at the edge of the movement.

Push your pelvis forwards

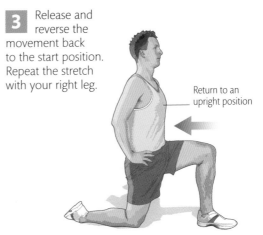

3 Release and reverse the movement back to the start position. Repeat the stretch with your right leg.

Return to an upright position

HIP CIRCLE

This rotational dynamic stretch offers a useful warm-up for your core muscles. In contrast to the torso rotation (**»p.48**) you should keep your upper body stationary while rotating your hips.

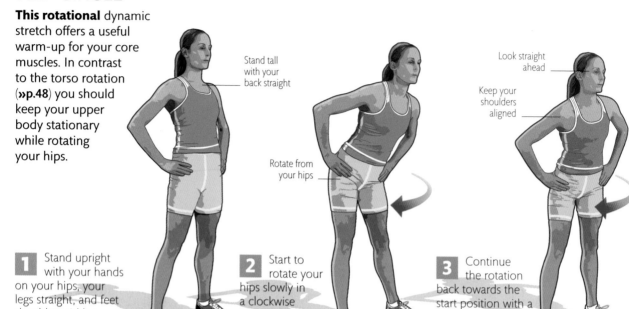

Stand tall with your back straight

Rotate from your hips

Look straight ahead

Keep your shoulders aligned

1 Stand upright with your hands on your hips, your legs straight, and feet shoulder-width apart.

2 Start to rotate your hips slowly in a clockwise direction. Keep your back straight.

3 Continue the rotation back towards the start position with a smooth, controlled movement.

CHILD'S POSE

This movement gently mobilizes your spine and hips while also working your shoulders and upper back. If you find the exercise uncomfortable, you can place a rolled-up towel between the back of your thighs and calves. To increase the stretch, reach your hands in front of you as far as you can.

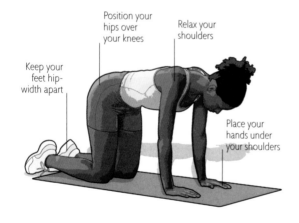

Position your hips over your knees

Relax your shoulders

Keep your feet hip-width apart

Place your hands under your shoulders

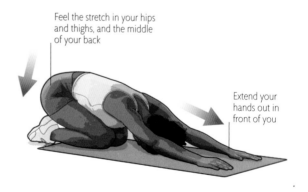

Feel the stretch in your hips and thighs, and the middle of your back

Extend your hands out in front of you

1 Kneel on all fours with your hands in line with your shoulders, your fingers pointing forwards, and your knees directly below your hips. Keep your back and neck straight.

2 Keeping your hands in position, slowly lower yourself down onto your heels until your forehead touches the mat. Extend your hands in front of you as far as is comfortable.

COBRA EXTENSION

This simple exercise is designed to stretch and strengthen your lower back muscles and improve your spinal flexibility. You should aim to perform the movement with a slow, fluid motion, keeping your neck and shoulders relaxed throughout.

SCORPION STRETCH

This is an excellent all-body stretch that improves your spinal flexibility. The movement can take some practice, but good technique is key, so focus on achieving the correct position rather than trying to push the stretch too far.

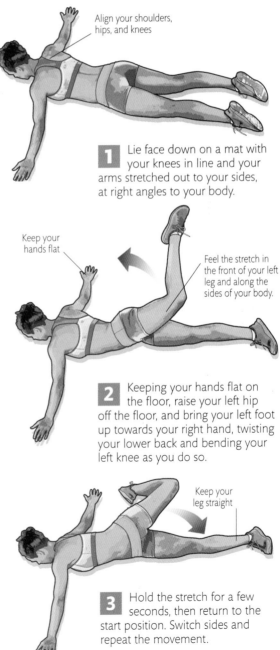

Align your shoulders, hips, and knees

1 Lie face down on a mat with your knees in line and your arms stretched out to your sides, at right angles to your body.

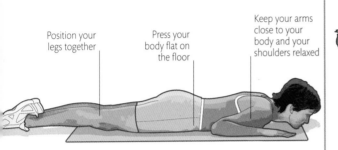

Position your legs together

Press your body flat on the floor

Keep your arms close to your body and your shoulders relaxed

1 Lie face down on a mat with your hands flat on the floor and roughly level with your chin. Extend your feet, keeping your legs together. Breathe in.

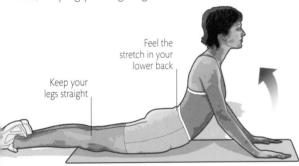

Feel the stretch in your lower back

Keep your legs straight

Keep your hands flat

Feel the stretch in the front of your left leg and along the sides of your body.

2 Pressing your hips against the mat and breathing out, lift your torso upwards slowly, using your arms for support. Raise your head and shoulders as high as you can, keeping your lower back relaxed.

2 Keeping your hands flat on the floor, raise your left hip off the floor, and bring your left foot up towards your right hand, twisting your lower back and bending your left knee as you do so.

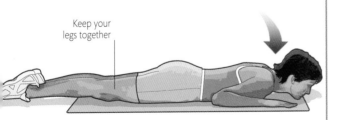

Keep your legs together

Keep your leg straight

3 Pause briefly at the top of the movement, then lower your torso back to the start position with a smooth, controlled movement, and using your arms for support.

3 Hold the stretch for a few seconds, then return to the start position. Switch sides and repeat the movement.

BACK ROLL

This dynamic stretch is an excellent way of mobilizing the muscles of your spine, lower back, and buttocks. Aim to perform the movement with a slow, controlled movement, and use a mat to cushion your spine as you roll. Be careful not to place strain on your neck.

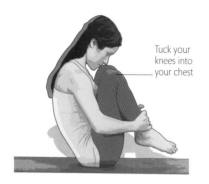

Tuck your knees into your chest

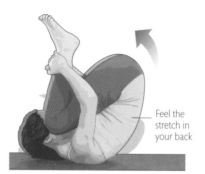

Feel the stretch in your back

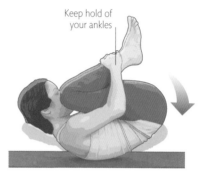

Keep hold of your ankles

1 Sit upright on a mat with your knees drawn up to your chest and your feet lifted off the floor. Engage your core, grip your ankles, and relax your neck, keeping your head facing forwards.

2 Gently roll backwards until your shoulder blades are resting on the floor, with your knees tucked up to your chest. Keep your core engaged and be careful not to roll onto your neck.

3 Hold the stretch for a few seconds, then reverse the movement with a smooth, controlled motion, rolling forwards to return to the start position.

SKIER

This excellent mobilizing stretch works your spine and shoulder joints in one fluid movement. It also encourages your upper and lower body to function as a unit. The exercise requires good co-ordination and range of motion, so it may take some practice to perfect.

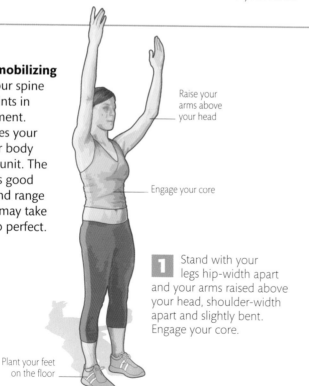

Raise your arms above your head

Engage your core

Plant your feet on the floor

1 Stand with your legs hip-width apart and your arms raised above your head, shoulder-width apart and slightly bent. Engage your core.

2 Bending your knees and dropping your buttocks back into a half squat, swing your upper body down and forwards, keeping your arms straight, your core engaged, and your back in a neutral position.

Keep your arms straight and your elbows soft

STANDING ROLL-DOWN

This dynamic stretch helps to mobilize the muscles of your lower back, while providing additional benefits to your hamstrings and shoulders. You should perform the exercise with a smooth, fluid movement.

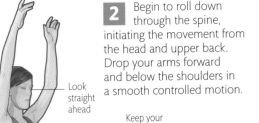

2 Begin to roll down through the spine, initiating the movement from the head and upper back. Drop your arms forward and below the shoulders in a smooth controlled motion.

3 Continue the movement until you are as fully folded through the spine and hips as possible, without straining. Relax your head, neck, and shoulders. Hold briefly, then return to start position in a slow, fluid motion.

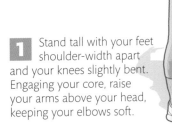

Look straight ahead

Keep your core muscles engaged

Allow a gentle arch in the middle of your back

Support your back using your core

Keep your head down and your shoulders relaxed

1 Stand tall with your feet shoulder-width apart and your knees slightly bent. Engaging your core, raise your arms above your head, keeping your elbows soft.

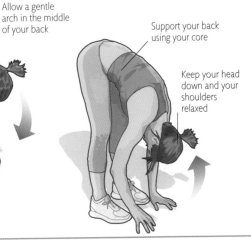

3 Remaining in the half-squat position, continue the swinging movement with your arms outside your legs, keeping your arms straight and your elbows soft.

4 Keeping your arms straight, continue the swinging movement of your arms hands past your knees and towards your hips.

5 Extend the swing back and upwards, rotating at your shoulders until your arms are roughly parallel with your thighs. Pause briefly at the edge of the movement, then reverse the sequence to the start position.

Maintain the half-squat position

Keep your core engaged

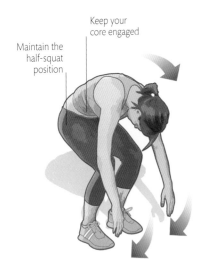

Rotate at your shoulders

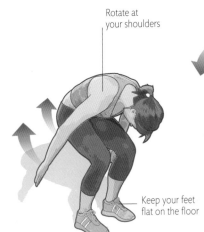

Keep your feet flat on the floor

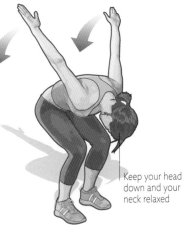

Keep your head down and your neck relaxed

ACTIVATION

Activation is a fundamental part of core training, helping to strengthen your core and prevent injuries. The "deep" core muscles responsible for stabilization are not as easy to feel as "surface" muscles, and engaging them therefore requires time, focus, and control. Concentrate on your breathing and technique to ensure you are performing the movements correctly.

ACTIVE PELVIC FLOOR

TARGET MUSCLES	TARGET MOVEMENT
■ Transverse abdominis	
■ Pelvic floor	
■ Multifidus	

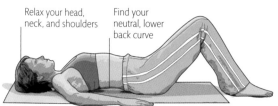

Isometric

DIFFICULTY LEVEL

This exercise gently stretches the muscles and ligaments of your back, strengthening your core and improving your posture; it also helps relieve pressure on your facet joints. You should perform this exercise on the floor at first, but as your technique improves you can try it standing up.

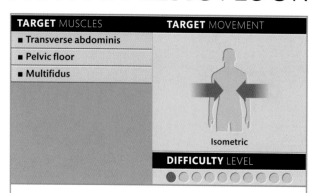

Deltoids

External obliques

Rectus abdominis

Internal obliques (deep)

Transverse abdominis (deep)

Pectorals

Multifidus (deep)

Pelvic floor (deep)

Erector spinae (hidden)

Quadratus lumborum (deep)

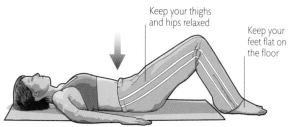

Relax your head, neck, and shoulders

Find your neutral, lower back curve

1 Lie on your back with your knees bent at a comfortable angle, your feet flat on the floor and hip-width apart, your arms by your sides, and your lower back in a neutral arch. Relax in this position before you begin.

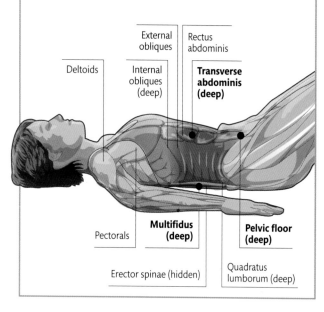

Keep your thighs and hips relaxed

Keep your feet flat on the floor

2 Gently press the small of your back into the floor and tilt your pubic bone upwards by engaging your abdominal and pelvic floor muscles. Hold for at least three seconds.

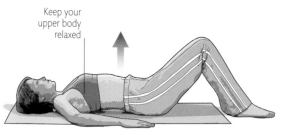

Keep your upper body relaxed

3 Relax and return to the start position, so that the small of your back is slightly arched once more. Repeat as required and relax.

PROGRESSION 1

This kneeling pelvic tilt helps if you have poor posture or a back complaint. Some experts recommend this as an alternative for the supine version of the exercise (left) because it gives you a greater range of movement.

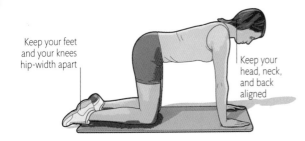

Keep your feet and your knees hip-width apart

Keep your head, neck, and back aligned

1 Kneel on a mat with your hands under your shoulders and your knees under your hips, keeping your back in a neutral position, and breathe in deeply.

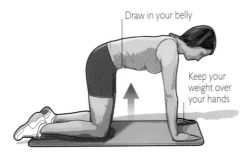

Draw in your belly

Keep your weight over your hands

2 Breathe out, pulling your abdominals in tight, and suck in your belly button towards your spine. With one fluid motion, reverse the curve in your lower back and tilt your hips.

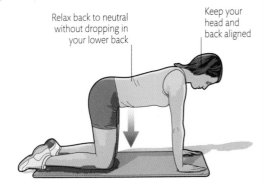

Relax back to neutral without dropping in your lower back

Keep your head and back aligned

3 Release your spine to a neutral position, without dropping through your back. Inhale and exhale, feeling the movement within your abs. Repeat as required.

PROGRESSION 2

It is harder to perform the pelvic tilt in an upright posture, either standing or sitting, but doing this movement on an exercise ball provides a helpful guide, as the ball will shift forwards slightly when you do the exercise correctly.

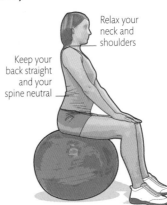

Relax your neck and shoulders

Keep your back straight and your spine neutral

1 Sit up straight on an exercise ball, with your feet parallel and hip-width apart. Rest your hands on your knees. Keep your back straight and your spine neutral. Breathe in deeply, maintaining this position.

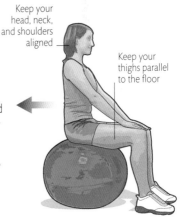

Keep your head, neck, and shoulders aligned

Keep your thighs parallel to the floor

2 Exhale forcefully, pulling your abdominals in tight and drawing them in towards your spine. With one fluid motion, reverse the curve in your lower back by tucking your hips under your torso and rolling the ball forward very slightly as you do so.

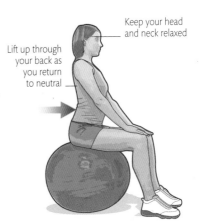

Keep your head and neck relaxed

Lift up through your back as you return to neutral

3 Hold the position for a few seconds, then release to return to the neutral position in step 1. Repeat as required and relax.

PILLOW SQUEEZE

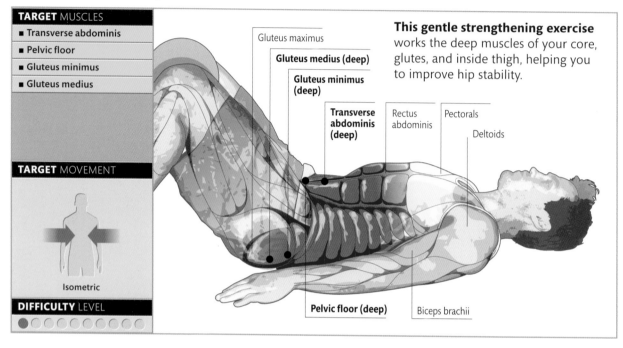

TARGET MUSCLES
- Transverse abdominis
- Pelvic floor
- Gluteus minimus
- Gluteus medius

TARGET MOVEMENT

Isometric

DIFFICULTY LEVEL

Gluteus maximus

Gluteus medius (deep)

Gluteus minimus (deep)

Transverse abdominis (deep)

Rectus abdominis

Pectorals

Deltoids

Pelvic floor (deep)

Biceps brachii

This gentle strengthening exercise works the deep muscles of your core, glutes, and inside thigh, helping you to improve hip stability.

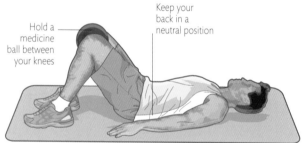

Hold a medicine ball between your knees

Keep your back in a neutral position

1 Place a medicine ball between your knees and lie on your back with your pelvis in a neutral position. With your feet flat on the ground, bend your knees at a right angle.

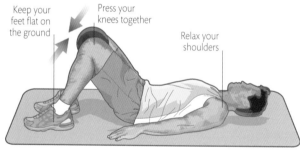

Keep your feet flat on the ground

Press your knees together

Relax your shoulders

2 Squeeze your knees together as hard as is comfortable. Hold the position for 5 seconds, engaging all core muscles, then relax to the start position. Repeat as required.

PROGRESSION 1

Raising your knees off the ground adds instability to the movement. Lie on your back with your pelvis in a neutral position and a medicine ball between your knees. With feet together, lift your knees up until at a right angle with your hips. Hold the position for 5 seconds, then relax.

PROGRESSION 2

This version of the exercise makes your core and glutes work harder because the squeeze is positioned further away from your hips. With a rolled-up towel between your feet, lie on your front with forehead resting on the back of your hands, and your legs straight. Brace your abdomen and keep your buttocks tight. Squeeze the inside of your feet together. Hold for 5 seconds, then relax to the start position.

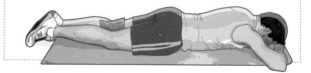

HEEL SLIDE

TARGET MUSCLES

- Transverse abdominis
- Internal obliques
- Pelvic floor
- Multifidus
- Quadratus lumborum

TARGET MOVEMENT

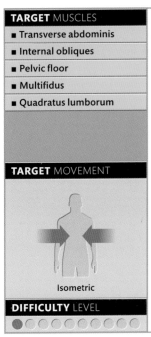

Isometric

DIFFICULTY LEVEL

This exercise is good for improving your awareness and stability of neutral hip and lower spinal alignment and helps to strengthen the deep core muscles that support it.

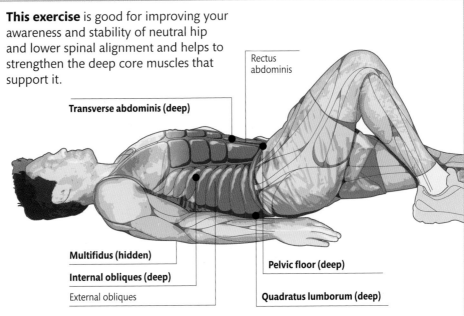

Rectus abdominis

Transverse abdominis (deep)

Multifidus (hidden)

Internal obliques (deep)

External obliques

Pelvic floor (deep)

Quadratus lumborum (deep)

1 Lie on your back with your legs stretched out straight in front of you, your arms by your sides, and your heels pressed lightly against the floor. Locate your neutral hip and spine position before you begin this exercise.

2 Slowly bend your right knee up by sliding your right heel along the ground. Bend it as far as you can without rocking or lifting your hips off the ground, or disturbing the lumbar spine position. Keep your core engaged throughout.

3 Slide your right leg back to the start position, without allowing the hips to rock to one side. Stay weighted in the tailbone and keep your core engaged. Alternate with each leg for the required number of reps, then relax.

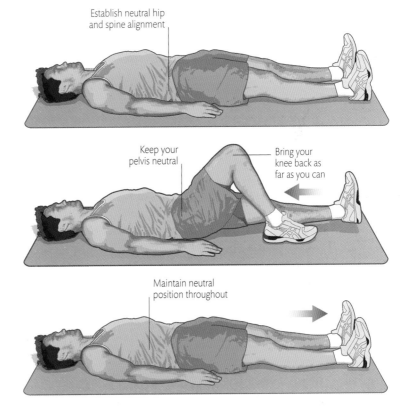

Establish neutral hip and spine alignment

Keep your pelvis neutral

Bring your knee back as far as you can

Maintain neutral position throughout

KNEE FOLD

TARGET MUSCLES	TARGET MOVEMENT
■ Transverse abdominis	
■ Internal obliques	
■ Pelvic floor	
■ Hip flexors	
■ Multifidus	

Isometric

DIFFICULTY LEVEL

This is a moderate-impact core-stabilizing exercise that helps to strengthen the deep muscles of your abdomen and your lower back. It can also be a useful exercise for preventing pain in your lumbar region. To get the best results from the exercise, keep the muscles of your core engaged throughout.

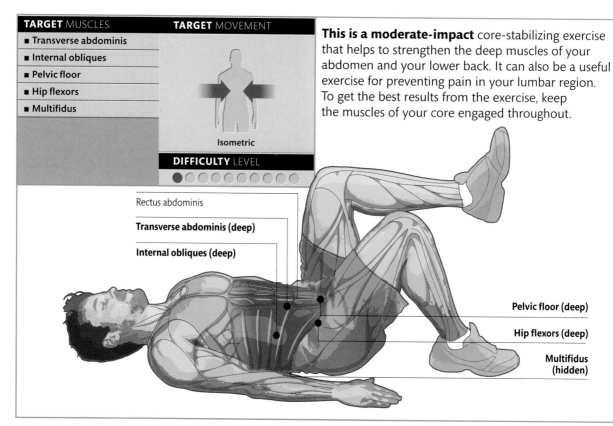

Rectus abdominis

Transverse abdominis (deep)

Internal obliques (deep)

Pelvic floor (deep)

Hip flexors (deep)

Multifidus (hidden)

VARIATION

This simple version of the movement keeps one foot anchored on the floor at all times – use this variation if you need a gentle warm-up, or if you want to try a less demanding version of the exercise. Keep your core engaged throughout and concentrate on maintaining good form.

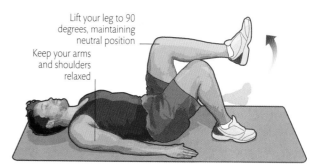

Brace your abdomen

Align your feet and knees at hip-width

Plant your feet flat on the ground

Lift your leg to 90 degrees, maintaining neutral position

Keep your arms and shoulders relaxed

1 Lie on your back with your spine and hips in a neutral position. Relax your upper back and shoulders, bend your knees, and engage your core.

2 Lift your left leg so that your hip and knee are at right angles, while maintaining hip and lower-back alignment. Hold this position for a few seconds, then slowly lower your legs to the start position. Repeat as required, then switch legs.

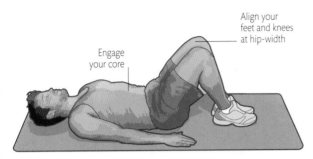

Engage your core

Align your feet and knees at hip-width

1 Lie on your back and bend your knees, with your feet flat on the floor. Relax your shoulders and upper back, engage your core, and keep your spine and hips in a neutral position.

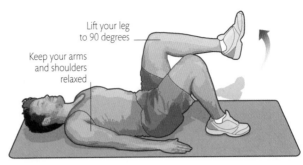

Lift your leg to 90 degrees

Keep your arms and shoulders relaxed

2 Keeping your core engaged, lift your left leg so that your hip and knee are at right angles. Keep your right foot on the floor and maintain neutral position.

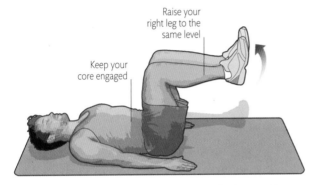

Raise your right leg to the same level

Keep your core engaged

3 With your core engaged, lift your right leg until it is level with your left. Hold this position for a few seconds; avoid tilting your hips and dropping your back.

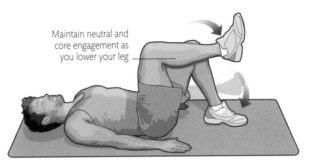

Maintain neutral and core engagement as you lower your leg

4 Keeping your core engaged, slowly lower your left leg until your left foot is flat on the floor, without letting your lower back arch, then lower your right leg.

PROGRESSION

Once you have mastered the basic exercise, try this more demanding progression, in which you raise both legs at once. Focus on maintaining core stability and neutral alignment throughout the movement. Keep your core engaged and your knees bent at a consistent angle, and avoid dropping or over-arching through your lower back.

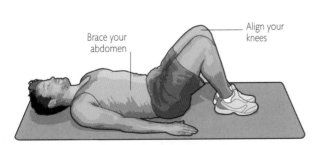

Brace your abdomen

Align your knees

1 Lie flat on your back, relaxing your upper back and shoulders, and with your spine in a neutral position. Bend your knees, while keeping your feet flat on the floor at all times.

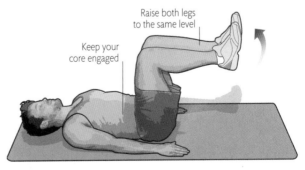

Raise both legs to the same level

Keep your core engaged

2 Engage your core. Lift both legs off the floor, keeping them aligned and hold neutral spine alignment. Hold this position for a few seconds, then slowly lower your legs to the start position without letting your lower back lift.

TOE TAP

TARGET MUSCLES	TARGET MOVEMENT
■ Transverse abdominis	
■ Internal obliques	
■ Pelvic floor	
■ Multifidus	
■ Quadratus lumborum	Isometric

DIFFICULTY LEVEL

This is a moderate-impact core-stabilizing exercise that can be helpful for strengthening the deep muscles of your abdomen and lower back. To get the best results from the movement, ensure you keep your core engaged throughout.

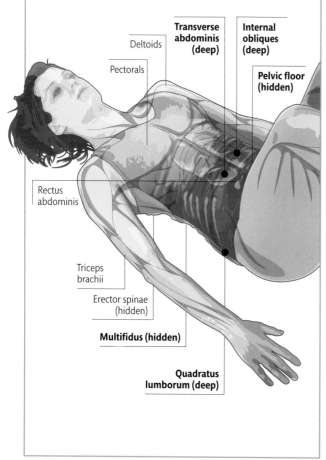

Deltoids

Transverse abdominis (deep)

Internal obliques (deep)

Pectorals

Pelvic floor (hidden)

Rectus abdominis

Triceps brachii

Erector spinae (hidden)

Multifidus (hidden)

Quadratus lumborum (deep)

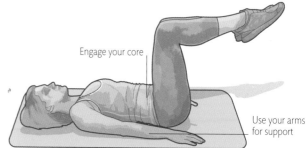

Engage your core

Use your arms for support

1 Lie on your back with your arms by your side. Engage the core and lift your legs in the air with your knees and feet at hip width. Keeping your spine and hips in a neutral position, relax your shoulders, using your arms to stabilize you if you need to.

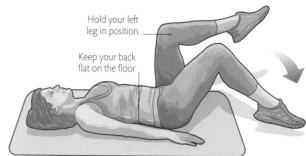

Hold your left leg in position

Keep your back flat on the floor

2 Keeping your core engaged, and holding your left leg at a right angle, lower your right leg towards the floor slowly and with control, without letting your back arch off the floor.

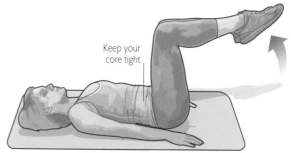

Keep your core tight

3 Hold at the edge of the movement, keeping your core braced, then return to the start position, maintaining control as you do so. Repeat as required, then swap legs.

PROGRESSION 1

Once you have mastered the basic movement you can make it harder by performing the exercise with both legs at the same time. This works the muscles of the abdomen and lower back much more intensely.

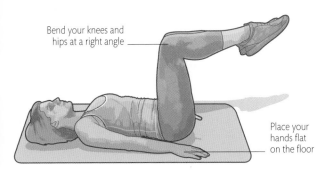

Bend your knees and hips at a right angle

Place your hands flat on the floor

1 Lie on your back with your arms by your sides. Bracing your abdomen, lift your legs into the air with your knees and feet together, and your toes pointing out. Use your arms to stabilize yourself if necessary.

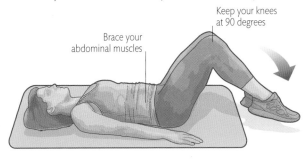

Keep your knees at 90 degrees

Brace your abdominal muscles

2 Keeping your core engaged, slowly lower both feet under control, without letting them drop to the floor.

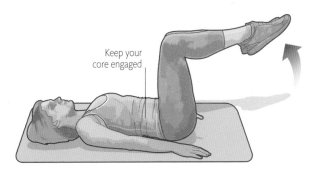

Keep your core engaged

3 Hold at the edge of the movement, then return to the start position, slowly and with good control.

PROGRESSION 2

Raising your arms off the floor adds an element of instability, making your core work even harder. Adopt the same starting position as in Progression 1, but raise your arms straight up. Keeping your arms still, and your core tight, alternately lower each foot to the floor.

PROGRESSION 3

The alternating movement of this progression adds the challenge of lateral instability. Begin with your arms vertical and your feet off the floor, knees bent. Lower your left arm and left leg to the floor at the same time. Return to the starting position, repeat as required, and switch sides.

PROGRESSION 4

This progression adds dynamic movement and rotational instability. Begin with your arms vertical and your feet off the floor, knees bent. Lower your left arm behind you, drawing your left knee to your chest, and extending your right leg as far as possible without arching your back. Repeat as required. Swap sides.

PRONE ABDOMINAL HOLLOWING

TARGET MUSCLES
- Transverse abdominis
- Pelvic floor
- Multifidus

This simple exercise helps you to develop good strength and control of your pelvic floor, transverse abdominis, and spinal stabilizing muscles. Gradually increase the number of repetitions as you progress.

TARGET MOVEMENT

Isometric

DIFFICULTY LEVEL

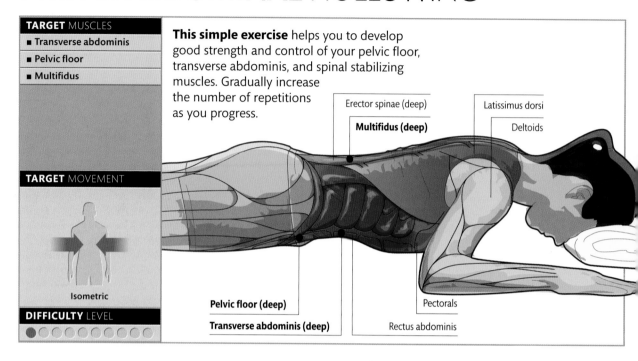

Erector spinae (deep)

Multifidus (deep)

Latissimus dorsi

Deltoids

Pelvic floor (deep)

Transverse abdominis (deep)

Pectorals

Rectus abdominis

1 Lie face down on a mat with a small towel beneath your head. Position your arms beside you, pointing forwards, palms down, your elbows bent at right angles. Reach forwards with the top of your head to lengthen your spine, keeping your shoulders apart. Breathe in deeply.

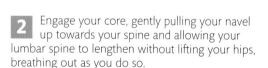

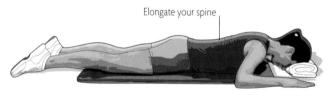

Elongate your spine

2 Engage your core, gently pulling your navel up towards your spine and allowing your lumbar spine to lengthen without lifting your hips, breathing out as you do so.

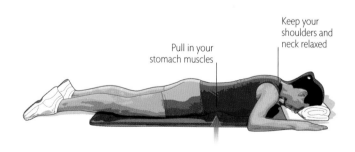

Pull in your stomach muscles

Keep your shoulders and neck relaxed

3 Hold your abdomen in for 5 seconds, then inhale as you return to the start position in a slow, controlled movement. Repeat as required.

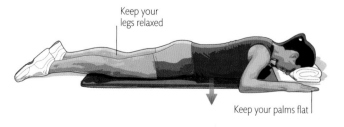

Keep your legs relaxed

Keep your palms flat

DART

TARGET MUSCLES

- Transverse abdominis
- Pelvic floor
- Erector spinae
- Multifidus
- Quadratus lumborum
- Gluteus minimus
- Gluteus medius
- Gluteus maximus

TARGET MOVEMENT

Extension

DIFFICULTY LEVEL

This activation exercise encourages deep core stability and strengthens the muscles of your upper back and glutes. It is one of the most effective exercises for improving posture awareness and alignment.

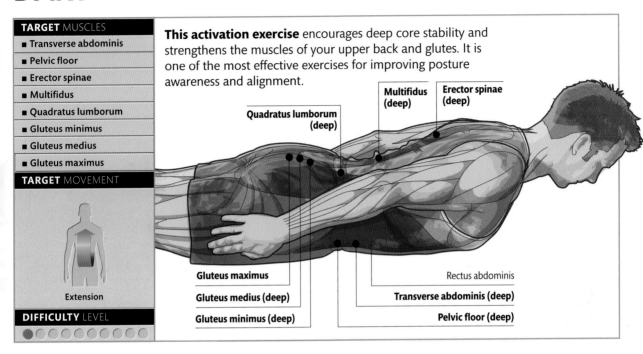

Multifidus (deep)

Erector spinae (deep)

Quadratus lumborum (deep)

Gluteus maximus

Gluteus medius (deep)

Gluteus minimus (deep)

Rectus abdominis

Transverse abdominis (deep)

Pelvic floor (deep)

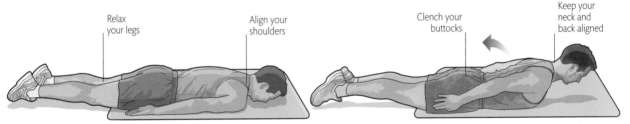

Relax your legs

Align your shoulders

Clench your buttocks

Keep your neck and back aligned

1 Lie face down on a mat, with your arms by your sides, palms up. Relax your trunk and legs. Breathe in, engaging your abdominals before you begin to move.

2 Lift your head, lengthening your neck. Raise your shoulders off the floor, rolling your palms in to face your thighs and draw your legs together to engage your glutes. Use your abs and lower back to control the movement.

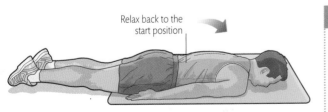

Relax back to the start position

3 Hold briefly, ensuring you maintain abdominal engagement, spinal length, and hip alignment, then return to the start position slowly and smoothly.

PROGRESSION

Once you have mastered the basic exercise, you can add a greater element of instability by placing a stability disc beneath your hips and lower abdomen. As before, control the movement using your glutes and the muscles of your lower back.

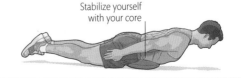

Stabilize yourself with your core

OYSTER

TARGET MUSCLES
■ Transverse abdominis
■ Pelvic floor
■ Multifidus
■ Gluteus medius
■ Gluteus maximus

TARGET MOVEMENT

Isometric

DIFFICULTY LEVEL

This exercise is a simple but excellent movement for working the deep, stabilizing muscles of your buttocks, improving your hip stability and alignment, while also building your overall core stability.

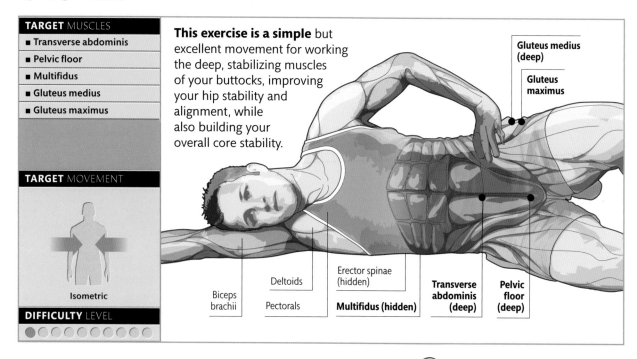

Gluteus medius (deep)

Gluteus maximus

Biceps brachii

Deltoids

Erector spinae (hidden)

Pectorals

Multifidus (hidden)

Transverse abdominis (deep)

Pelvic floor (deep)

1 Lie on your right side, bending both the hips and knees at a 45-degree angle. Extend your right arm so that it is in line with the body, and rest your head on it. Bend your left arm at the elbow and place the left hand on to the floor in front of you.

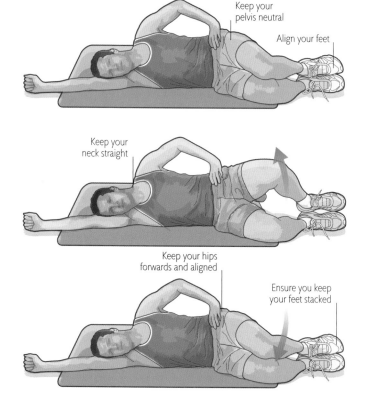

Keep your pelvis neutral

Align your feet

2 Keeping your neck straight, your hips and shoulders in line, and your feet touching, engage your core and begin lifting the knee of your left leg, rotating at your hip.

Keep your neck straight

3 Lift your left knee as far as it will go without straining, keeping your hips aligned. Slowly lower your knee back to the start position, and repeat for the required number of reps before swapping sides.

Keep your hips forwards and aligned

Ensure you keep your feet stacked

PRONE LEG LIFT

TARGET MUSCLES

- Transverse abdominis
- Internal obliques
- Pelvic floor
- Multifidus
- Quadratus lumborum
- Gluteus medius
- Gluteus maximus

TARGET MOVEMENT

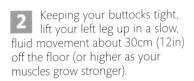

Isometric

DIFFICULTY LEVEL

This exercise strengthens the large muscles of your buttocks and helps to improve pelvic stability. Avoid using your back in the movement.

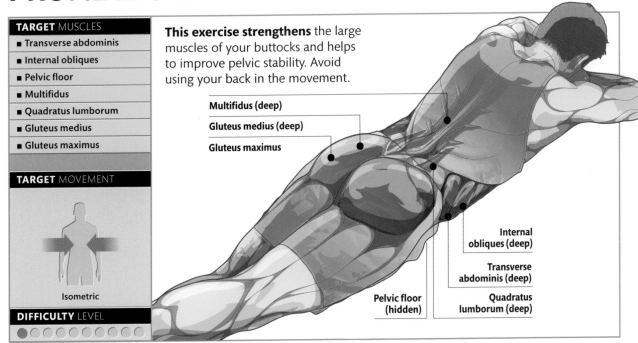

Multifidus (deep)

Gluteus medius (deep)

Gluteus maximus

Internal obliques (deep)

Transverse abdominis (deep)

Pelvic floor (hidden)

Quadratus lumborum (deep)

1 Lie on your front with your forehead resting on the back of your arms and your knees straight. Engage your core to support your back and squeeze your buttocks together.

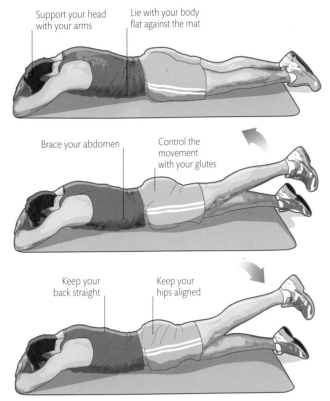

Support your head with your arms

Lie with your body flat against the mat

Brace your abdomen

Control the movement with your glutes

Keep your back straight

Keep your hips aligned

2 Keeping your buttocks tight, lift your left leg up in a slow, fluid movement about 30cm (12in) off the floor (or higher as your muscles grow stronger).

3 Pause at the top of the movement, then return to the start position, slowly and with control. Repeat the required number of reps, before switching legs.

STAR

TARGET MUSCLES

- Transverse abdominis
- Pelvic floor
- Erector spinae
- Multifidus
- Quadratus lumborum
- Gluteus medius
- Gluteus maximus

TARGET MOVEMENT

Isometric

DIFFICULTY LEVEL

This exercise is useful for stabilizing the muscles along your spine, while also strengthening the shoulders, lower back, and buttocks.

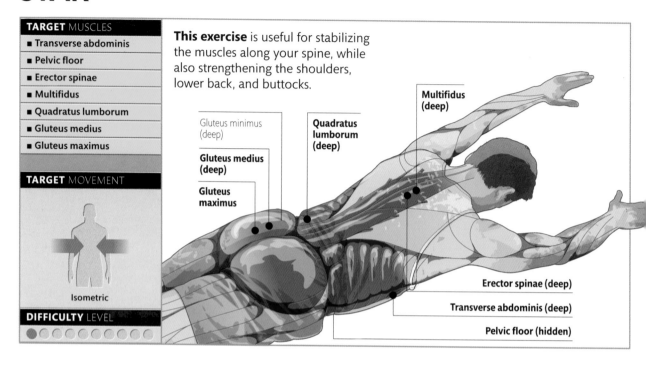

Gluteus minimus (deep)

Gluteus medius (deep)

Gluteus maximus

Quadratus lumborum (deep)

Multifidus (deep)

Erector spinae (deep)

Transverse abdominis (deep)

Pelvic floor (hidden)

1 Lie face down with your forehead resting on a mat. Align your neck and head. Extend your arms in front of you with the palms facing down. Lengthen your torso by stretching your neck away from your body, and engage your core.

Keep your feet together

Place your palms flat on the floor

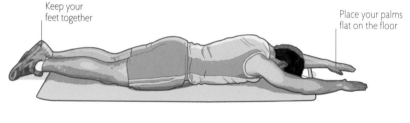

2 Keeping your head in line with your spine and your abs tight, raise the left arm and the right leg 8–15cm (3–6in) off the floor. Hold your glutes tight and avoid rocking your hips and dropping through your lower back.

Contract your glutes

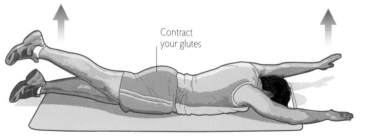

3 Hold the position briefly. Lower your limbs slowly and with control to return to the start position. Repeat as required and switch sides.

Use your glutes to stop your body from rotating

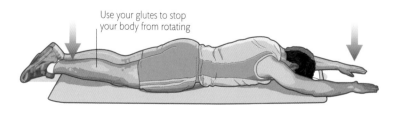

BACK EXTENSION

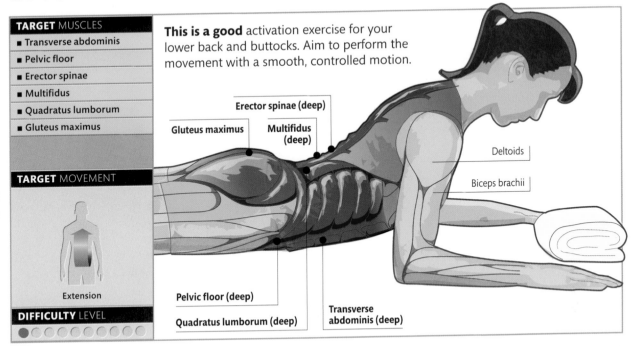

TARGET MUSCLES
- Transverse abdominis
- Pelvic floor
- Erector spinae
- Multifidus
- Quadratus lumborum
- Gluteus maximus

TARGET MOVEMENT

Extension

DIFFICULTY LEVEL

This is a good activation exercise for your lower back and buttocks. Aim to perform the movement with a smooth, controlled motion.

Erector spinae (deep)

Gluteus maximus

Multifidus (deep)

Deltoids

Biceps brachii

Pelvic floor (deep)

Quadratus lumborum (deep)

Transverse abdominis (deep)

1 Lie face down on a mat with a folded towel positioned under your forehead to ensure proper alignment of the head and neck with your spine. Bend your arms and rest your forearms on the floor, palms down. Breathe in deeply.

Align your head and neck with your spine

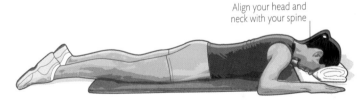

2 Engage your core and reach forwards with the top of your head to lengthen your spine, keeping your shoulders apart. Then, facing downwards, lift your head and shoulders off the floor, exhaling as you do so without using your arms.

Hold your glutes tight

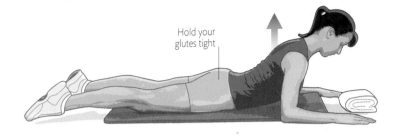

Keep your legs straight

3 Pause at the top of the movement, then inhale and return to the start position, slowly and with control.

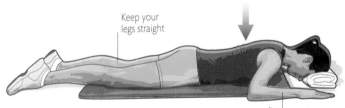

Keep your arms flat

SUPERMAN

TARGET MUSCLES

- Transverse abdominis
- Pelvic floor
- Multifidus
- Quadratus lumborum
- Gluteus medius
- Gluteus maximus

TARGET MOVEMENT

Isometric

DIFFICULTY LEVEL

This exercise strengthens the spinal extensor muscles and deep spinal stabilizers, which support your spine, and builds strength and stability in your buttocks, lower back, and shoulders.

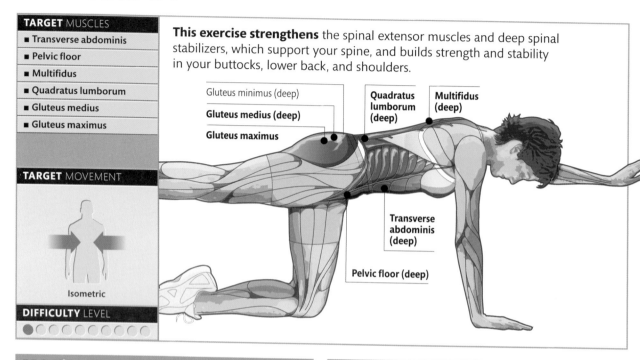

Gluteus minimus (deep)

Gluteus medius (deep)

Gluteus maximus

Quadratus lumborum (deep)

Multifidus (deep)

Transverse abdominis (deep)

Pelvic floor (deep)

PROGRESSION 1

Assuming the main position with a leg raised, rather than an arm, demands greater balance and core control, because it increases the level of rotational instability working your spinal stabilizers and deep core muscles. To perform the movement, engage your core and lift your right leg behind you to hip height. Balance and hold for 10 seconds, then return to the start position, then switch legs. Be sure to keep your back straight and your shoulders and hips aligned.

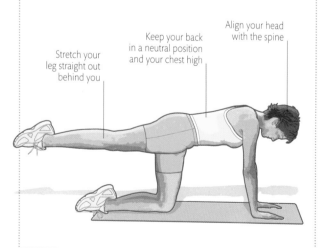

Stretch your leg straight out behind you

Keep your back in a neutral position and your chest high

Align your head with the spine

PROGRESSION 2

Combining an arm lift and a leg lift requires additional strength and stability as it increases rotational instability even more than removing the support of a leg. Contracting your abs, simultaneously lift your right leg behind you to hip height and your left arm forwards to shoulder height. Hold for 10 seconds, return to the start position, then repeat with your other leg and arm. Maintain a straight line from your shoulders to your hips throughout.

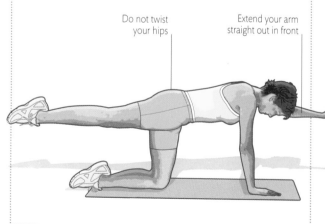

Do not twist your hips

Extend your arm straight out in front

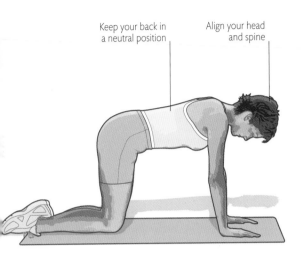

Keep your back in a neutral position

Align your head and spine

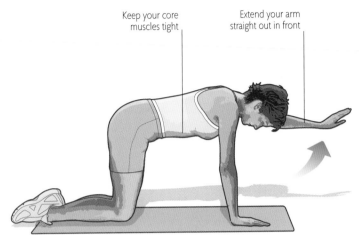

Keep your core muscles tight

Extend your arm straight out in front

1 Kneel on all fours, with your knees aligned squarely beneath your hips. Keep your back straight and position your hands directly beneath your shoulders, pressing them flat on the ground and pointing forwards.

2 Engaging your core, raise one arm in front of you. Hold for 10 seconds, then return to the start position. Repeat the movement with your other arm and relax to the start position.

PROGRESSION 3

Placing a stability disc beneath your supporting arm makes your core work even harder to stabilize your spine. Assume the same position as in the main sequence, kneeling with your feet hip-width apart, and your right hand on the stability disc. Supporting your body weight on your right arm and knees, extend your left arm up, keeping it in line with your torso. Hold this position, then lower your left arm, relax, and swap arms. Keep your core engaged, your shoulders and hips in line, and your spine in a neutral position.

PROGRESSION 4

Using the body position of Progression 2 but placing a stability disc beneath your supporting arm offers an even greater challenge to your core. With your feet hip-width apart, support your weight on your right arm. In one smooth, controlled movement, extend your right leg out straight behind you and reach your left arm out in front. Hold, then return to the start position and switch arms and legs. Maintain a straight line from your shoulders to your hips and keep your core tight throughout.

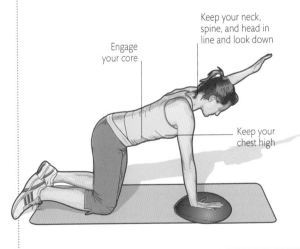

Keep your neck, spine, and head in line and look down

Engage your core

Keep your chest high

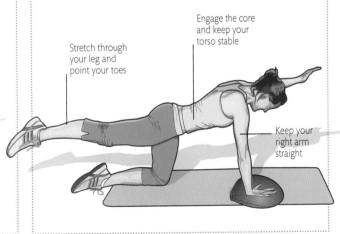

Engage the core and keep your torso stable

Stretch through your leg and point your toes

Keep your right arm straight

FOUNDATION

The exercises in this section are the building blocks of good core strength and stability. You should aim to master them before moving on to those in the Intermediate and Advanced sections. To ensure you get the best results, focus on performing each exercise correctly, maintaining good form throughout and controlling the movements with your core.

ABDOMINAL CRUNCH

TARGET MUSCLES	TARGET MOVEMENT
▪ Rectus abdominis	
▪ Transverse abdominis	
▪ Internal obliques	
▪ Pelvic floor	

Flexion

DIFFICULTY LEVEL

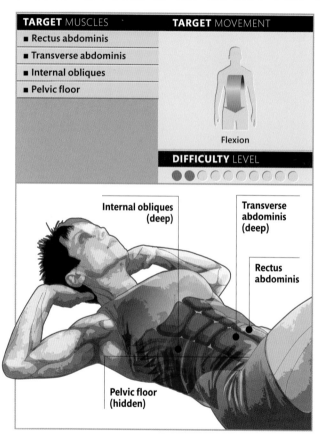

Internal obliques (deep)

Transverse abdominis (deep)

Rectus abdominis

Pelvic floor (hidden)

VARIATION

To work your abdominal area in a different way you can use a "pulsing" action. Pause at the top of the movement and slide your hands up and down your thighs. The movement of each pulse is very small, but aim to squeeze your abs a little bit tighter each time. Aim for around five pulses per crunch.

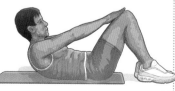

The basic abdominal crunch is one of the simplest and most popular of all core exercises. Good form is key – control the movement with your core and keep your shoulders and neck relaxed.

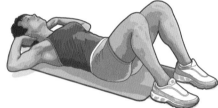

1 Lie on a mat with your knees bent, your feet flat on the floor, and your fingers against the sides of your head.

Keep your chin tucked in

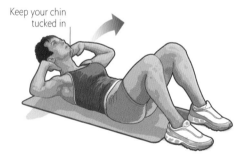

2 Crunching up from your core, lift your shoulders and upper back off the floor without straining.

Keep your hips stable throughout

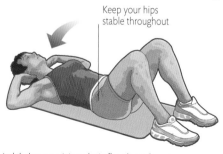

3 Hold the position briefly, then lower your upper body slowly to the floor, controlling the downward phase with your core.

PROGRESSION 1

Removing the support of your legs adds an element of instability, making the muscles of your core work a little harder as you perform the crunch. From the original start position, extend your legs straight into the air with your knees together. Using your abs, crunch up as far as you can, then hold briefly before returning to the start position slowly and under control.

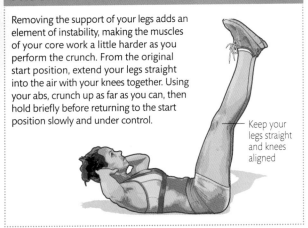

Keep your legs straight and knees aligned

PROGRESSION 2

Performing the exercise while holding a medicine ball increases the load on your abs, making the movement more challenging. Holding the ball firmly with both hands, assume the normal starting position, then raise the ball in the air with your arms straight. Hold the ball in this position while you carry out the desired number of repetitions.

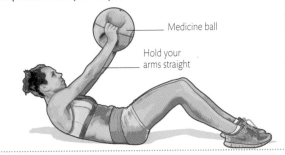

Medicine ball

Hold your arms straight

PROGRESSION 3

Resting your hips on an exercise ball requires good balance and stability. It makes it even harder for you to support your weight with your legs, because the ball can also move in any number of directions. To start, carefully lie back against the ball with your feet firmly planted on the floor and your knees bent at right angles. Crunch up with your upper body, hold, and return to the start position.

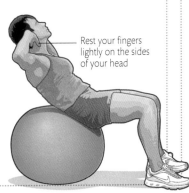

Rest your fingers lightly on the sides of your head

PROGRESSION 4

Positioning your feet on a bench works your core stabilizers harder and increases the range of movement. Lie on your back with your calves on the bench, so that your hips and knees are bent at right angles. Control the movement with your core, curling your torso towards your knees, and avoid "cheating" the movement by hooking your heels on the edge of the bench.

Keep your head straight

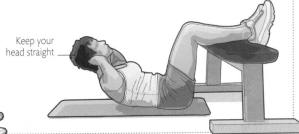

PROGRESSION 5

Using an unbalanced legs position introduces an element of lateral instability, which provides a further challenge to your core stabilizers. Lie with your back on the mat, and your hands across your chest. Straighten one leg along the floor and bend the other at 90 degrees with your foot flat on the floor. Crunch up with your abdominals to control the movement, pause at the edge of the movement, then return to the start position. Repeat as required and switch legs.

Keep one leg straight

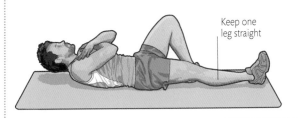

PROGRESSION 6

This even more challenging version of the movement involves a variation of the Progression 5 crunch – with your lower back resting on a stability disc to add even more instability. Lie at an angle with the disc under your lumbar spine and your hands crossed lightly on your chest. Control the crunch with your core, pause at the edge of the movement, before returning to the starting position. Repeat as required and change legs.

Control the movement with your core

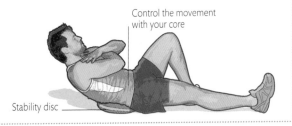

Stability disc

LEG CIRCLE

TARGET MUSCLES	**TARGET** MOVEMENT
■ Transverse abdominis	
■ Internal obliques	
■ Pelvic floor	
■ Multifidus	
■ Quadratus lumborum	
■ Gluteus minimus	
■ Gluteus medius	Isometric

DIFFICULTY LEVEL

This activation exercise is simple but demands good form and hip flexibility. Keep your pelvis and core stationary, and avoid rocking from side to side. Use your palms to brace yourself against the floor, and keep your head as still as possible.

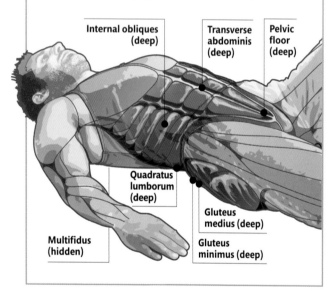

Internal obliques (deep)

Transverse abdominis (deep)

Pelvic floor (deep)

Quadratus lumborum (deep)

Gluteus medius (deep)

Multifidus (hidden)

Gluteus minimus (deep)

PROGRESSION 1

Carrying out the movement with a straight leg introduces an element of instability, making the core muscles work harder. Lie on your back in the start position and raise the left leg, keeping it straight. Rotate it in a clockwise circle, keeping your pelvis anchored. Repeat and switch sides.

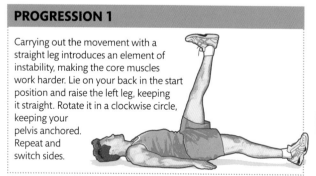

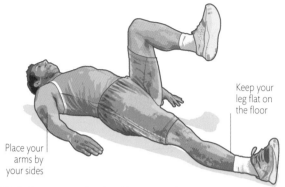

Keep your leg flat on the floor

Place your arms by your sides

1 Lie on your back with your palms on the floor. Raise your left leg with the knee bent at a 90-degree angle.

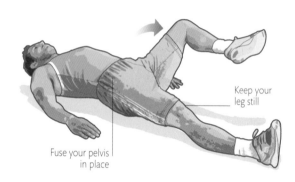

Keep your leg still

Fuse your pelvis in place

2 Rotate your left leg in a clockwise circle down and to the left, keeping your core engaged and your pelvis firmly anchored.

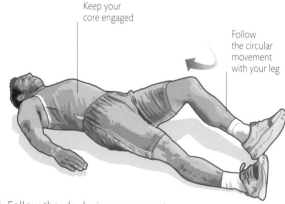

Keep your core engaged

Follow the circular movement with your leg

3 Follow the clockwise movement down to the bottom of the circle, keeping your left knee bent. Continue the movement around to the start position, repeat, and switch sides.

REVERSE CURL

TARGET MUSCLES	TARGET MOVEMENT

- Rectus abdominis
- Transverse abdominis
- Pelvic floor

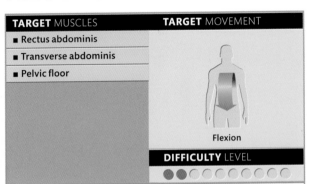

Flexion

DIFFICULTY LEVEL

This exercise works in a similar way to the crunch, but involves you moving your legs rather than your torso. It works your lower abs, without placing stress on your shoulders and neck, which are resting on the floor.

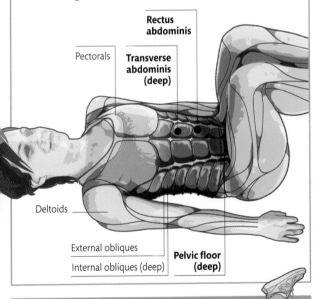

Pectorals

Rectus abdominis

Transverse abdominis (deep)

Deltoids

External obliques

Internal obliques (deep)

Pelvic floor (deep)

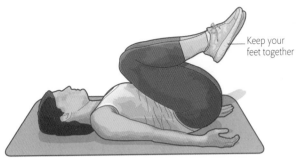

Keep your feet together

1 Lie down with your arms by your sides, palms up, and draw your knees up towards your chest, keeping your lower back flat and your shoulders relaxed. Engage your core.

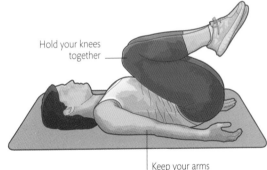

Hold your knees together

Keep your arms flat on the floor

2 Resting your head on the floor and keeping the back in a neutral position, draw your knees further in towards your chest in a crunching movement. Repeat this movement the desired number of times.

PROGRESSION 1

This progression of the basic exercise involves extending the movement to raise your legs and your torso off the ground. Because you have removed the support of your lower back, your core muscles have to work even harder to stabilize your body. Begin by lying on your back with your arms by your sides, palms pressed down for stability.

PROGRESSION 2

Once you have mastered Progression 1 you can make it even more challenging by holding an exercise ball between your legs. Perform the exercise in the same way as Progression 1, using your arms for support.

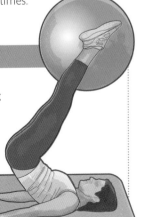

DORSAL RAISE

TARGET MUSCLES
■ Transverse abdominis
■ Pelvic floor
■ Erector spinae
■ Multifidus
■ Quadratus lumborum
■ Gluteus maximus

TARGET MOVEMENT

This simple exercise helps to strengthen the spinal stabilizing muscles of your lower back. Aim to perform the movement with good form and avoid jerking up with your shoulders, which can strain your neck.

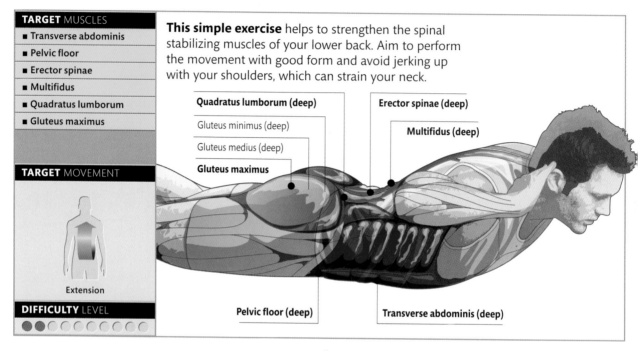

Quadratus lumborum (deep)

Gluteus minimus (deep)

Gluteus medius (deep)

Gluteus maximus

Erector spinae (deep)

Multifidus (deep)

Pelvic floor (deep)

Transverse abdominis (deep)

Extension

DIFFICULTY LEVEL

1 Lie face down with your legs together. Place your hands by the side of your head, keeping your shoulders relaxed and your core active. Breathe in.

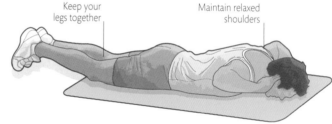

Keep your legs together

Maintain relaxed shoulders

2 Exhale as you lift your upper body off the floor. Perform the movement slowly, controlling it with your core. Be careful not to jerk your head or strain the muscles of your lower back or neck.

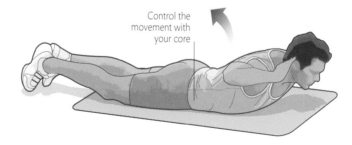

Control the movement with your core

3 Breathe in, hold briefly at the top of the movement, maintaining an active core, then slowly and gently lower yourself back to the start position.

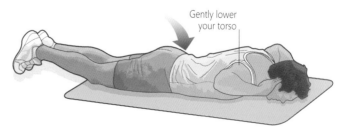

Gently lower your torso

PROGRESSION 1

Performing the dorsal raise with your arms extended increases the load on your core, making the deep muscles of your abdominals, back, and glutes work harder to stabilize your torso.

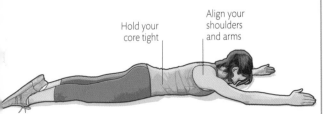

Hold your core tight

Align your shoulders and arms

1 Lie on your front with your legs together, and the top of your feet resting on the floor. Raise your arms above your head, with elbows soft, palms facing in, shoulders relaxed, and fingertips pointing forwards. Breathe in to prepare for the movement.

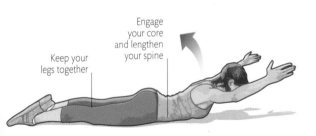

Keep your legs together

Engage your core and lengthen your spine

2 Engaging your core, breathe out as you lift the upper body off the floor. Keep your head and your upper body in line, and support from the abdominals to avoid over-extending in your lower back.

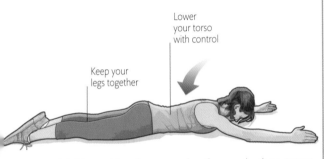

Lower your torso with control

Keep your legs together

3 Hold this position for a couple of seconds, then return to the start position slowly and with good control. Repeat the movement as required.

PROGRESSION 2

This further progression of the exercise involves raising both your arms and legs at the same time, removing the support of your legs and adding an even greater level of instability.

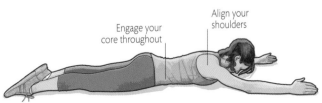

Engage your core throughout

Align your shoulders

1 Lie down on your front with your legs slightly apart and your feet resting on the floor. With elbows soft, palms facing in, and shoulder relaxed, stretch your arms out and forwards. Breathe in.

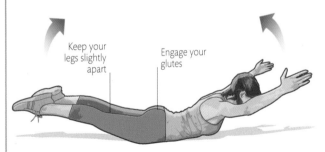

Keep your legs slightly apart

Engage your glutes

2 Engage your core and breathe out as you lift your upper body and legs off the floor. Keep your legs slightly apart and glutes engaged to help avoid over-extending the lower back.

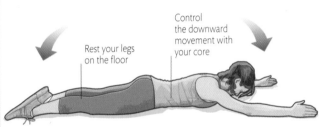

Control the downward movement with your core

Rest your legs on the floor

3 Hold this position for a couple of seconds, before lowering your arms and legs back to the start position. Repeat the movement as required.

SIT-UP

TARGET MUSCLES	TARGET MOVEMENT

- Rectus abdominis
- Transverse abdominis
- Internal obliques
- Pelvic floor
- Hip flexors
- Multifidus
- Quadratus lumborum

Flexion

DIFFICULTY LEVEL

The sit-up is a well-used and effective exercise for strengthening abdominals and increasing hip flexion. Focus on using your core to drive the movement, and avoid straining your neck.

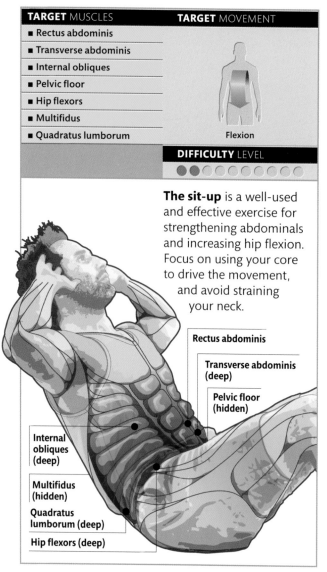

Rectus abdominis

Transverse abdominis (deep)

Pelvic floor (hidden)

Internal obliques (deep)

Multifidus (hidden)

Quadratus lumborum (deep)

Hip flexors (deep)

PROGRESSION

Changing the position of your arms alters the difficulty of the exercise. Extending your arms ahead of your knees provides the least resistance, while crossing your arms over your chest or holding them by your head increases difficulty. For an advanced workout, hold a weight plate to your chest.

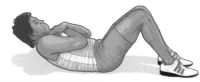

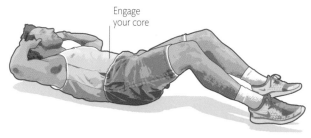

Engage your core

1 Lie on your back with your feet on the floor and your knees bent. Place the tips of your fingers on either side of your head.

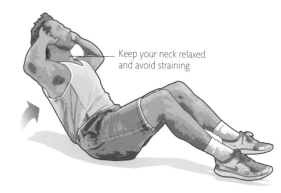

Keep your neck relaxed and avoid straining

2 Engage your core muscles and raise your torso upwards, leaving just your buttocks and feet on the floor. Drive the movement entirely with your core.

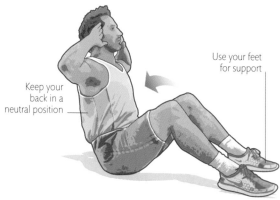

Keep your back in a neutral position

Use your feet for support

3 Pause at the edge of the movement, then slowly lower your upper body to the start position, controlling the movement with your core.

OBLIQUE CRUNCH

TARGET MUSCLES	TARGET MOVEMENT
■ Rectus abdominis	
■ Transverse abdominis	
■ External obliques	
■ Internal obliques	
■ Pelvic floor	

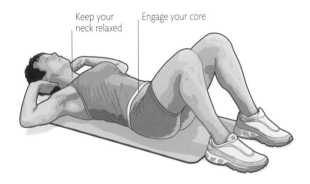

Rotation

DIFFICULTY LEVEL

This simple but effective core exercise works your obliques and transverse abdominis, building both rotational strength and the ability of your core to stabilize your spine and hips against external rotational forces.

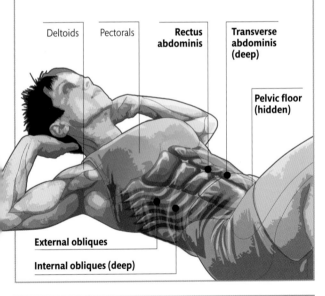

Deltoids · Pectorals · **Rectus abdominis** · **Transverse abdominis (deep)**

Pelvic floor (hidden)

External obliques

Internal obliques (deep)

PROGRESSION

Performing the movement on an exercise ball makes it harder because the ball can move in any number of directions. Carefully lie back on the ball with your legs hip-width apart. Crunch up and rotate from your upper body, hold, and return to the start position.

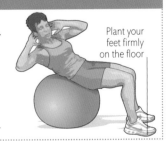

Plant your feet firmly on the floor

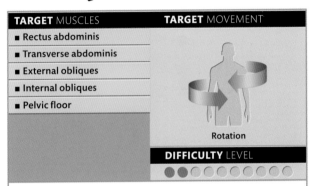

Keep your neck relaxed · Engage your core

1 Lie on a mat in neutral start position with your knees bent, your feet flat, and your fingers against the sides of your head. Breathe in.

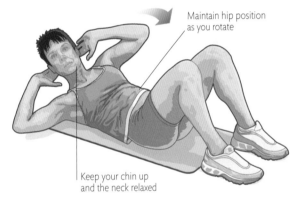

Maintain hip position as you rotate

Keep your chin up and the neck relaxed

2 Engage your core, exhale, and rotate your upper back off the floor aiming your left shoulder towards your right knee. Work from your abdominals, keeping the hips still.

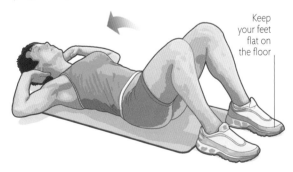

Keep your feet flat on the floor

3 Hold for a moment then lower your upper body slowly to the floor, using your core to control the movement.

SIDE-LYING LATERAL CRUNCH

TARGET MUSCLES	TARGET MOVEMENT
■ Rectus abdominis	
■ Transverse abdominis	
■ External obliques	
■ Internal obliques	
■ Pelvic floor	
■ Multifidus	
■ Quadratus lumborum	Side Flexion

DIFFICULTY LEVEL

This exercise improves your strength and core stability, and targets your external and internal obliques, improving trunk stability and side flexion. To avoid straining your neck, ensure that you support your head with your hand and control the movement using the core. For maximum effect, perform the movement slowly.

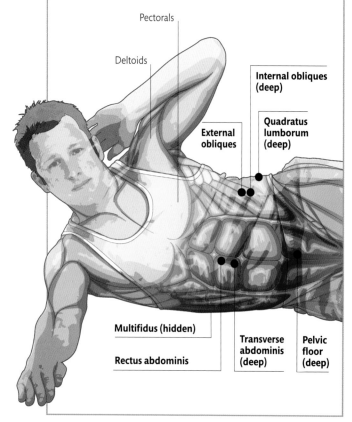

Pectorals

Deltoids

Internal obliques (deep)

Quadratus lumborum (deep)

External obliques

Multifidus (hidden)

Rectus abdominis

Transverse abdominis (deep)

Pelvic floor (deep)

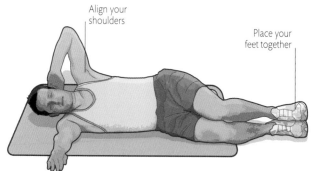

Align your shoulders

Place your feet together

1 Lie on your right side, with your right arm outstretched, palm down, and your left hand lightly supporting your head. Bend slightly from the waist so that your legs are at an angle of around 30 degrees to your torso.

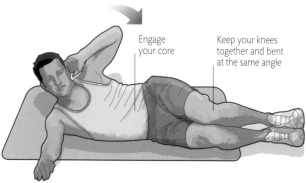

Engage your core

Keep your knees together and bent at the same angle

2 Squeeze your oblique muscles to raise your head and shoulders, taking care not to force the movement.

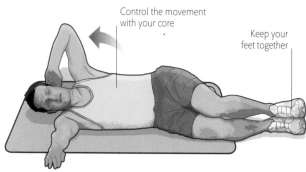

Control the movement with your core

Keep your feet together

3 Pause briefly at the top of the movement, then return to the start position slowly and under control. Complete the desired number of reps, then switch sides.

SIDE BEND

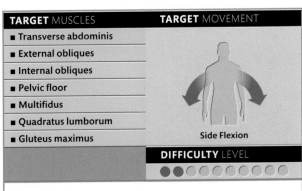

TARGET MUSCLES	TARGET MOVEMENT
■ Transverse abdominis	
■ External obliques	
■ Internal obliques	
■ Pelvic floor	
■ Multifidus	
■ Quadratus lumborum	
■ Gluteus maximus	Side Flexion

DIFFICULTY LEVEL

This exercise is a simple but effective way of strengthening your obliques, and stabilizing your spine against lateral and rotational forces. Practice with a light weight until you have perfected the movement – focus on controlling the upward and downward phases with your core, rather than using your arms to raise and lower the dumbbell.

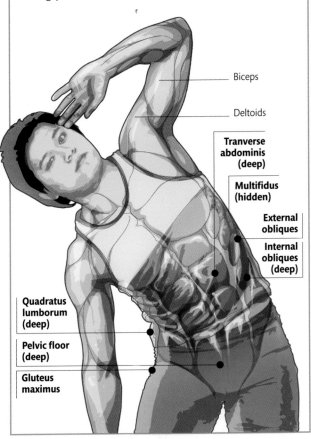

Biceps

Deltoids

Tranverse abdominis (deep)

Multifidus (hidden)

External obliques

Internal obliques (deep)

Quadratus lumborum (deep)

Pelvic floor (deep)

Gluteus maximus

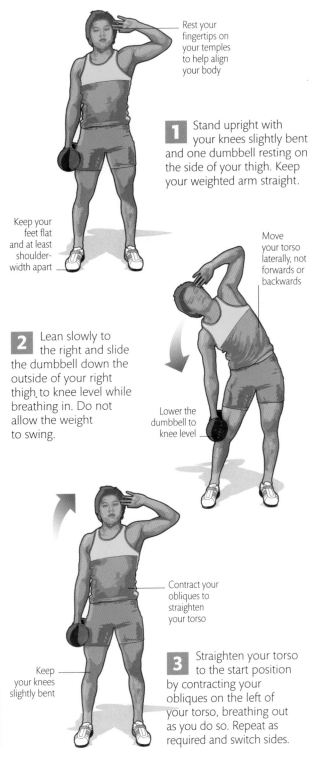

Rest your fingertips on your temples to help align your body

1 Stand upright with your knees slightly bent and one dumbbell resting on the side of your thigh. Keep your weighted arm straight.

Keep your feet flat and at least shoulder-width apart

Move your torso laterally, not forwards or backwards

2 Lean slowly to the right and slide the dumbbell down the outside of your right thigh to knee level while breathing in. Do not allow the weight to swing.

Lower the dumbbell to knee level

Contract your obliques to straighten your torso

Keep your knees slightly bent

3 Straighten your torso to the start position by contracting your obliques on the left of your torso, breathing out as you do so. Repeat as required and switch sides.

HEEL REACH

TARGET MUSCLES
- Rectus abdominis
- Transverse abdominis
- External obliques
- Internal obliques
- Pelvic floor
- Multifidus
- Quadratus lumborum

TARGET MOVEMENT

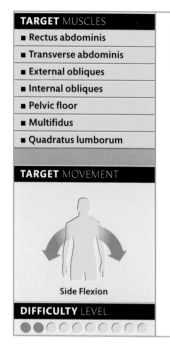

Side Flexion

DIFFICULTY LEVEL

This side flexion exercise works your obliques, improving trunk stability and control. Good form is key – ensure that you control the movements with your core.

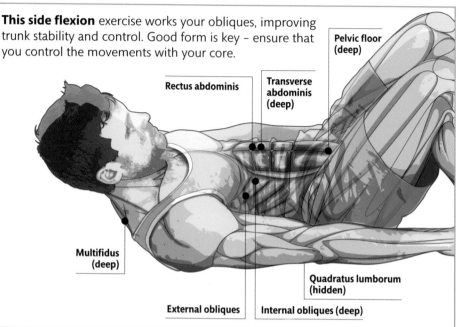

Pelvic floor (deep)

Rectus abdominis

Transverse abdominis (deep)

Multifidus (deep)

Quadratus lumborum (hidden)

External obliques

Internal obliques (deep)

1 Lie on your back with your arms by your sides, palms down, and bend the knees. Engage your core to raise your shoulders and upper back off the floor, keeping your neck relaxed and your spine in a neutral position.

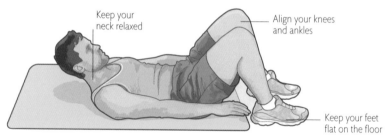

Keep your neck relaxed

Align your knees and ankles

Keep your feet flat on the floor

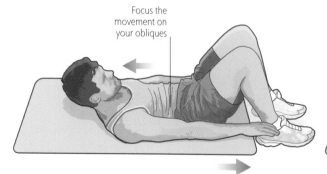

Focus the movement on your obliques

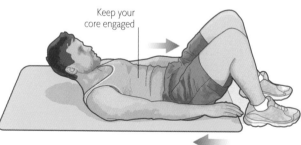

Keep your core engaged

2 Reach down as far as you can towards your right foot with your right hand in a slow and controlled movement, crunching the left side of your abdomen to drive the movement and avoid straining with your neck.

3 Pause briefly, then return to the starting position and alternate for the required number of repetitions. Repeat the movement to the left side of your body.

ROMAN CHAIR SIDE BEND

TARGET MUSCLES

- Transverse abdominis
- External obliques
- Internal obliques
- Pelvic floor
- Multifidus
- Quadratus lumborum
- Gluteus maximus

TARGET MOVEMENT

Side Flexion

DIFFICULTY LEVEL

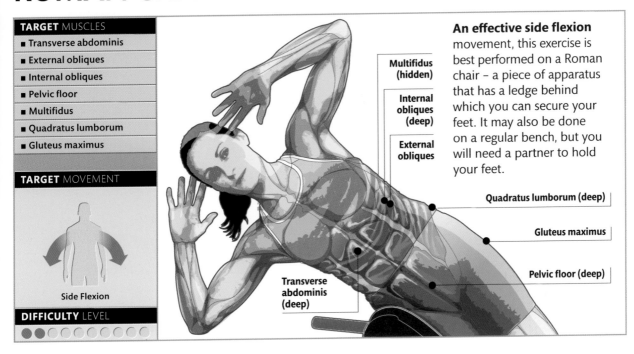

Multifidus
(hidden)

Internal
obliques
(deep)

External
obliques

Quadratus lumborum (deep)

Gluteus maximus

Pelvic floor (deep)

Transverse
abdominis
(deep)

An effective side flexion movement, this exercise is best performed on a Roman chair – a piece of apparatus that has a ledge behind which you can secure your feet. It may also be done on a regular bench, but you will need a partner to hold your feet.

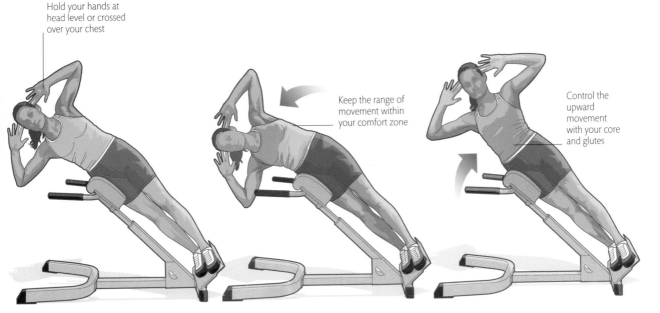

Hold your hands at head level or crossed over your chest

Keep the range of movement within your comfort zone

Control the upward movement with your core and glutes

1 Lie sideways on the Roman chair; adjust it so that your upper body can pivot comfortably at your hips towards the floor.

2 Lean slowly sideways towards the floor as far as is comfortable, taking care not to lean forwards or back. Breathe in on your descent.

3 Pause at the edge of the movement, then gently raise your body to the start position. Repeat as required and switch sides.

SIDE-LYING LEG LIFT

TARGET MUSCLES
- Transverse abdominis
- Internal obliques
- Pelvic floor
- Multifidus
- Quadratus lumborum
- Gluteus minimus
- Gluteus medius

TARGET MOVEMENT

Isometric

DIFFICULTY LEVEL

This exercise strengthens and stabilizes your core against lateral movements, while also working your glutes and hip flexors to improve your core control and balance.

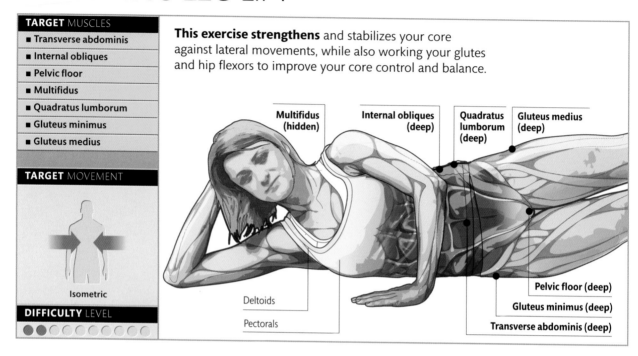

Multifidus (hidden)

Internal obliques (deep)

Quadratus lumborum (deep)

Gluteus medius (deep)

Pelvic floor (deep)

Gluteus minimus (deep)

Transverse abdominis (deep)

Deltoids

Pectorals

1 Lie on the right side of your body with your ankles stacked. Use the right hand to support your head, and place your left hand flat on the floor in front of you to help you stabilize.

2 Keeping your spine aligned, use the muscles of your core and upper legs to lift up your feet. Keep your feet stacked, and ensure your legs are aligned with your back.

3 Pause at the edge of the movement, then lower your feet slowly back to the start position. Repeat as required, then switch sides.

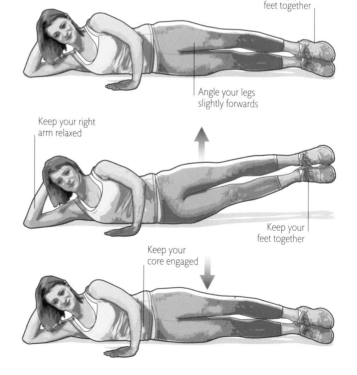

Keep your feet together

Angle your legs slightly forwards

Keep your right arm relaxed

Keep your feet together

Keep your core engaged

VARIATION

The side-lying leg kick offers a gentle balance exercise that also stretches the tendons in your legs, and provides a low-intensity workout for your core and arm muscles. Be careful on hard floors, or anywhere that might cause discomfort to your hips and elbows – use a mat if necessary. Remember to use slow, controlled movements when kicking your leg, and try to avoid placing any strain on the muscles of your neck while carrying out the desired number of repetitions.

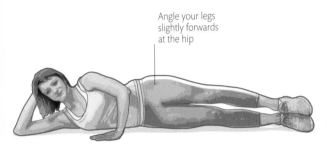

Angle your legs slightly forwards at the hip

1 Lie on your right side with your ankles together. Plant your left hand flat on the floor in front of you to help you stabilize, and support your head with your right hand.

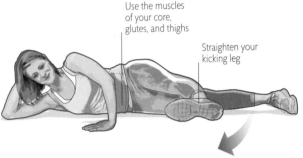

Use the muscles of your core, glutes, and thighs

Straighten your kicking leg

2 Keeping your upper body still, kick your left leg forwards as far as you can, using the muscles of your core and upper legs to control the movement.

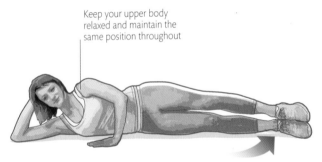

Keep your upper body relaxed and maintain the same position throughout

3 Briefly hold the position before swinging your left leg back through the start position, controlling the movement with the muscles of your core and thighs.

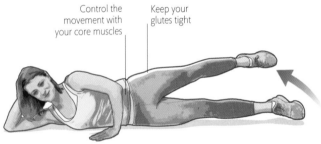

Control the movement with your core muscles

Keep your glutes tight

4 Swing your left leg back as far as you can, keeping the movement as smooth and controlled as possible, and holding your upper body in position.

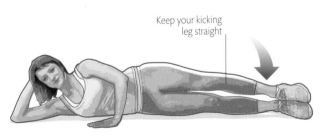

Keep your kicking leg straight

5 Pause at the edge of the movement, then swing your left leg forwards to return to the start position. Repeat the sequence as required, before switching legs.

PROGRESSION

Placing a stability disc beneath your hip adds an element of instability, making the muscles of your core work harder to balance your body as you perform the movement. Follow the same steps in the main sequence and repeat as necessary, before switching sides.

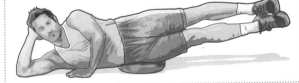

OBLIQUE REACH

TARGET MUSCLES

- Rectus abdominis
- Transverse abdominis
- External obliques
- Internal obliques
- Pelvic floor
- Hip flexors
- Multifidus
- Quadratus lumborum

TARGET MOVEMENT

Rotation

DIFFICULTY LEVEL

This simple but effective rotational core exercise works most of the muscles of your "abdominal girdle" (**»p.56**), responsible for posture. The twisting movement involved particularly challenges your internal and external obliques and helps you increase your ability to stabilize your spine against rotational forces. It is important to ensure that you focus the movements on your core to get the best results.

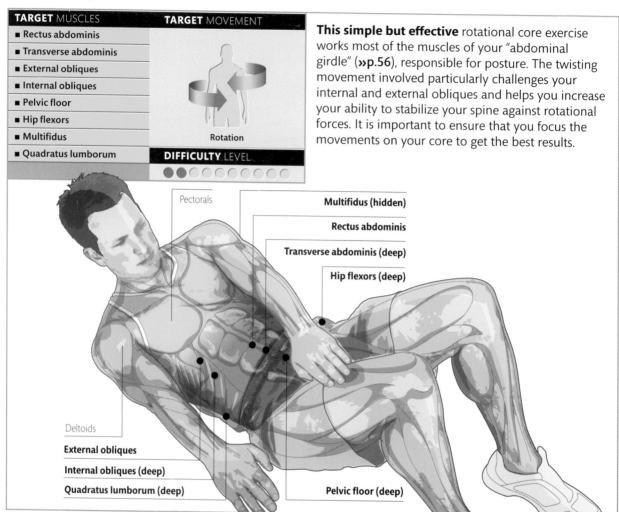

Pectorals

Multifidus (hidden)

Rectus abdominis

Transverse abdominis (deep)

Hip flexors (deep)

Deltoids

External obliques

Internal obliques (deep)

Quadratus lumborum (deep)

Pelvic floor (deep)

PROGRESSION 1

You can use a kettlebell to increase the load on your abdominal muscles. Grasp the weight in both hands and carry out the exercise as normal, controlling the movement with your core.

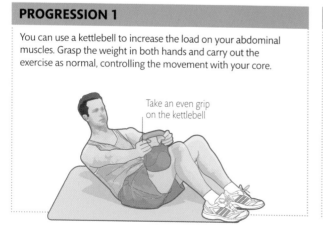

Take an even grip on the kettlebell

PROGRESSION 2

To increase the load on your abdominal muscles even further, replace the kettlebell with a medicine ball. Grasp the ball in both hands and carry out the exercise as normal.

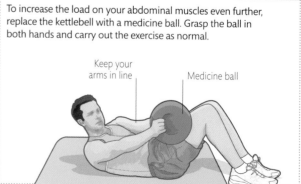

Keep your arms in line

Medicine ball

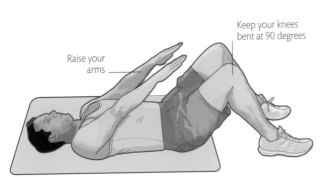

1 Lie on your back and raise your arms in front of you, palms down, fingers pointing to your knees. Lift your arms, then engage your core to raise your shoulders and upper back slightly, keeping the spine in a neutral position.

Raise your arms

Keep your knees bent at 90 degrees

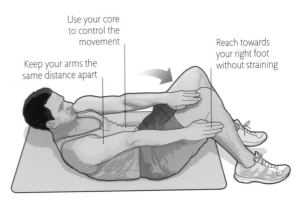

Use your core to control the movement

Keep your arms the same distance apart

Reach towards your right foot without straining

2 Reach as far as you can towards your right foot with both hands in a slow and controlled movement. Use your core muscles to drive the movement, crunching the right side of your abdomen to avoid straining with your neck.

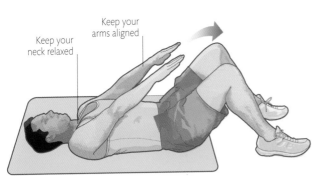

Keep your neck relaxed

Keep your arms aligned

3 Hold the position briefly, then slowly curl back to the horizontal, controlling the movement with your core. Keep your arms raised and slightly apart, and your knees bent at an angle of 90 degrees.

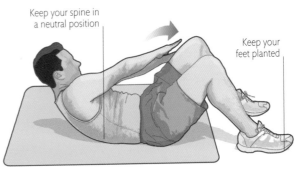

Keep your spine in a neutral position

Keep your feet planted

4 Switching the movement to the left side of your body, reach down as far as you can towards your left foot with both hands, crunching the left side of the abdomen. Hold the position briefly, then return to the start position.

PROGRESSION 3

Lifting your feet off the floor to perform the movement makes your core muscles work harder to stabilize your body. Bend your knees and hold them together, keeping your calves roughly parallel to the ground. Perform both phases of the movement under good control.

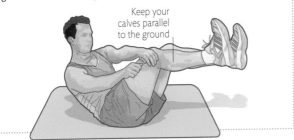

Keep your calves parallel to the ground

PROGRESSION 4

For an even more challenging exercise, perform the movement in Progression 3, but holding a kettlebell. Grasping a light kettlebell in both hands, carry out the exercise as normal, controlling movement with your core. Increase the weight as your strength increases.

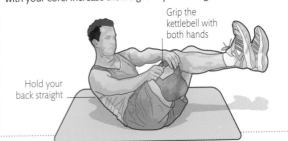

Grip the kettlebell with both hands

Hold your back straight

HIP ROLL

TARGET MUSCLES
■ Transverse abdominis
■ External obliques
■ Internal obliques
■ Pelvic floor
■ Hip flexors
■ Multifidus
■ Quadratus lumborum
■ Gluteus minimus
■ Gluteus medius

TARGET MOVEMENT

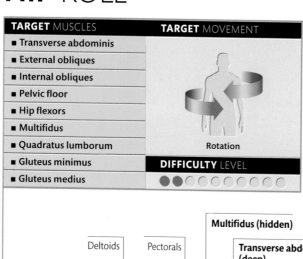

Rotation

DIFFICULTY LEVEL

This exercise strengthens your abdominals and lower back, as well as improving the general mobility of your lower and mid-back. While carrying out the movement, it is important to focus on keeping your upper back and shoulders in a consistent, stable position, in order to avoid rolling the whole body from side to side when you move your legs and hips. To begin with, you may find it helpful to use your outstretched arms to brace against the floor, and to find a point on the ceiling on which to fix your gaze to avoid moving your head.

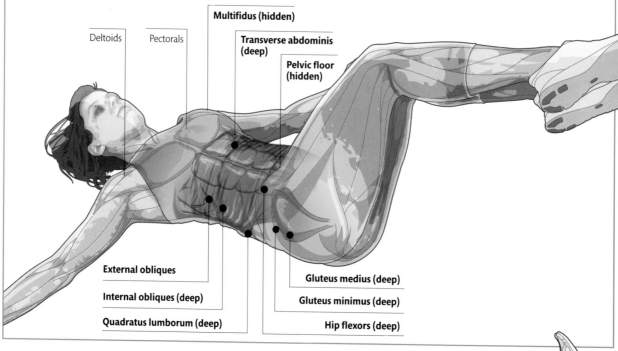

Multifidus (hidden)

Deltoids   Pectorals

Transverse abdominis (deep)

Pelvic floor (hidden)

External obliques

Internal obliques (deep)

Quadratus lumborum (deep)

Gluteus medius (deep)

Gluteus minimus (deep)

Hip flexors (deep)

VARIATION

This easier version of the exercise improves the mobility of your hips in a less challenging way. Bend your knees and place your feet on the floor, then gently roll the hips to the left and to the right, keeping your upper back flat. Repeat as needed, then return to the start position.

Keep your knees bent

Engage your core

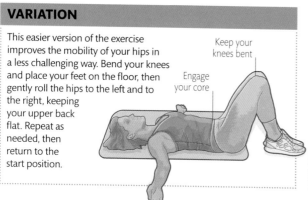

PROGRESSION 1

This progression makes your glutes and hip flexors work harder because it requires you to keep your legs straight throughout. In the start position, raise your legs straight up in the air and, keeping your lower back in neutral, roll your hips to your left and right, controlling the movement from your core.

Keep your legs straight

Engage your core

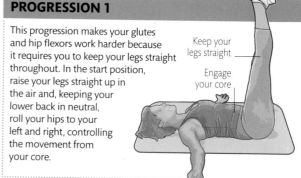

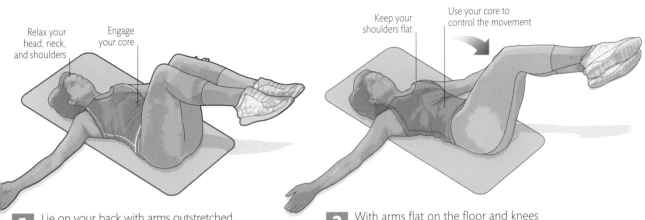

Relax your head, neck, and shoulders

Engage your core

Keep your shoulders flat

Use your core to control the movement

1 Lie on your back with arms outstretched, palms up. Raise your legs to 90 degrees, with knees together. Keep your core engaged and your lower back in a neutral position.

2 With arms flat on the floor and knees together, lift your right hip and roll your hips and legs to the left. Stop before your upper back begins to lift. Hold for a few seconds.

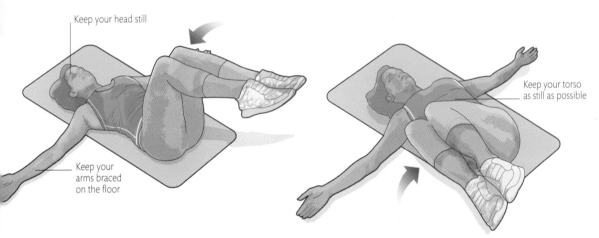

Keep your head still

Keep your arms braced on the floor

Keep your torso as still as possible

3 Initiating from your core, roll your hips and legs back to the centre, regaining your neutral position.

4 In the same way, roll your hips to the right, keeping your core engaged and using your arm for stability. Hold briefly, then return to start.

PROGRESSION 2

This progression removes the support of the arms, increasing the demands on your core, as you have to work harder to stabilize your body. Lie on your back, then raise your legs and arms straight up into the air. Roll your hips to your left and right, controlling the movement from your core. Repeat as required, then relax.

Keep your arms still

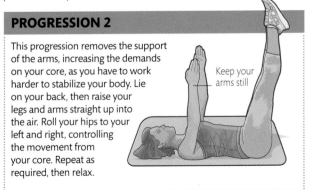

PROGRESSION 3

Introducing a medicine ball increases the work on your glutes and hip flexors, and engages the hip adductor and the muscles of your inner thigh. In the start position, grip a medicine ball with your knees, and roll your hips to the left and right.

Keep your back flat

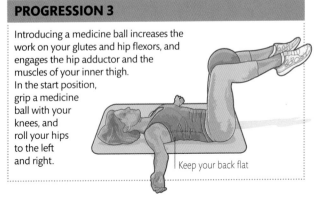

ROLL-BACK

TARGET MUSCLES	TARGET MOVEMENT
■ Rectus abdominis	
■ Transverse abdominis	
■ Internal obliques	
■ Pelvic floor	
■ Gluteus minimus	
■ Gluteus medius	Flexion

DIFFICULTY LEVEL

This exercise is excellent for spinal mobility, and for improving the stability, control, and strength of your abdominals and lower back. Aim for smooth movement, using the muscles of your core to control the downward roll.

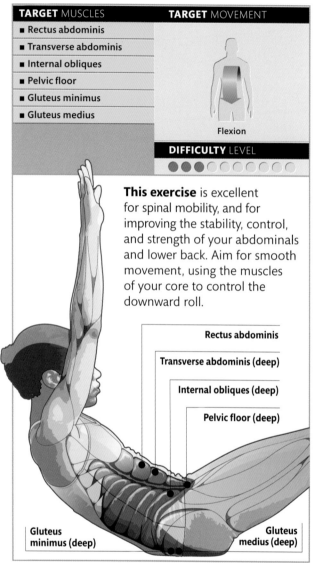

Rectus abdominis

Transverse abdominis (deep)

Internal obliques (deep)

Pelvic floor (deep)

Gluteus minimus (deep)

Gluteus medius (deep)

VARIATION

This easier version of the exercise uses the same basic starting position, but reduces your range of movement. Hold your thighs for support, as shown, and roll back so that only the small of your back lies flat against the floor. Hold the position before drawing yourself upright again.

Keep your elbows wide and your hips tucked

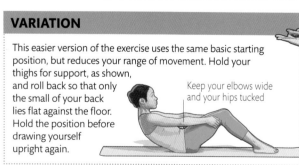

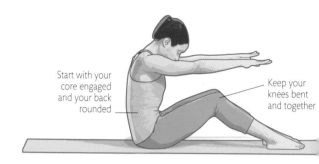

Start with your core engaged and your back rounded

Keep your knees bent and together

1 Start seated, contracting your abdominals and gently rounding your spine. Keep your feet flat on the floor, with your arms out in front of you and your shoulders relaxed.

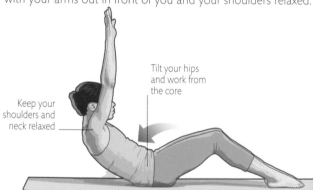

Tilt your hips and work from the core

Keep your shoulders and neck relaxed

2 Tilt your hips, tucking your tailbone, and begin to roll slowly backwards, using your abs to control the movement. Keeping your arms straight, continue rolling back, until the back of the hips and lower back are on the floor, encouraging your lower back and hip flexors to release.

Find a neutral spine position

3 Roll down all the way, elongating your spine as you do so. Find a neutral spine position, pause, then return to the start position. Control the movement with your core, rather than allowing your arms or momentum to jerk you up.

ROLL-UP

TARGET MUSCLES	TARGET MOVEMENT
■ Rectus abdominis	
■ Transverse abdominis	
■ Internal obliques	
■ Pelvic floor	
■ Gluteus minimus	
■ Gluteus medius	

Flexion

DIFFICULTY LEVEL

●●●●○○○○○○○

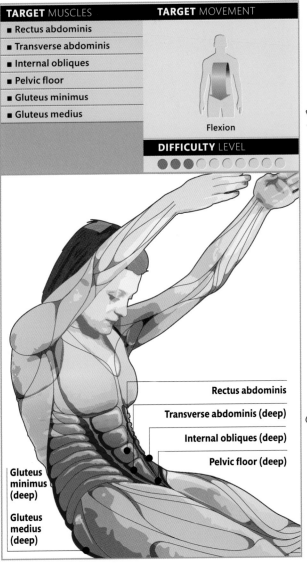

Rectus abdominis

Transverse abdominis (deep)

Internal obliques (deep)

Pelvic floor (deep)

Gluteus minimus (deep)

Gluteus medius (deep)

VARIATION

This easier version of the exercise, uses a half-sitting position to reduce your range of movement. Holding the back of your thighs, draw yourself into an upright position, controlling the movement with your core. Hold and return to the start position.

Hold your elbows wide and draw in your navel

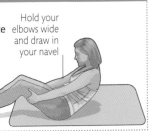

This exercise – a reverse of the roll-back (**left**) – helps to build strength in your core and requires good control of your abdominals and hip stabilizers. Avoid the temptation to "swing" yourself up with your upper body, and focus on using your core muscles.

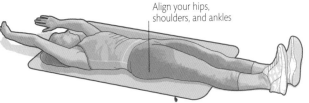

Align your hips, shoulders, and ankles

1 Lie on your back in a neutral hip and spine position, with your legs flat against the floor and your arms stretched out straight above your head. Engage the core to begin the movement.

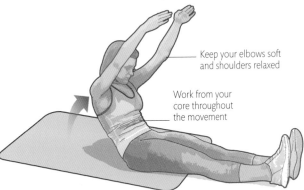

Keep your elbows soft and shoulders relaxed

Work from your core throughout the movement

2 Draw in your abdominals and nod your head to initiate the movement. Use the muscles of your core to roll you up slowly and with control. Keep your legs flat together and avoid pulling from your hip flexors.

Keep your abdominals contracted and your back rounded

Keep your legs relaxed

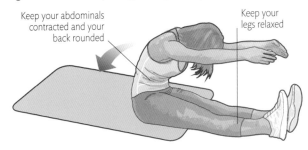

3 Continue the movement, stretching your fingertips towards your toes. Hold for a few seconds, then slowly lower yourself back to the starting position.

V LEG-RAISE

TARGET MUSCLES
- Rectus abdominis
- Transverse abdominis
- Pelvic floor
- Hip flexors

TARGET MOVEMENT

Flexion

DIFFICULTY LEVEL

This exercise provides a powerful workout for your abdominals and hip flexors; you can boost the intensity further by placing a weight between both your ankles. Ensure that the platform or bench you use is sufficiently stable.

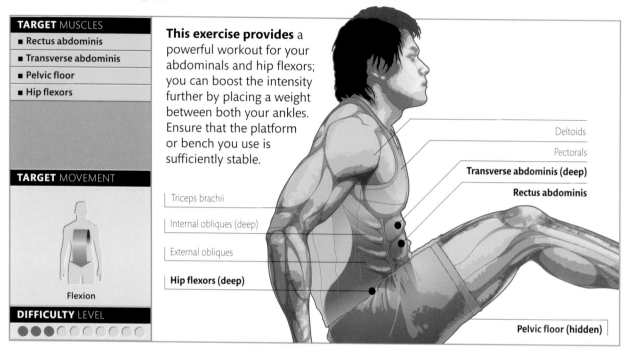

Deltoids

Pectorals

Transverse abdominis (deep)

Rectus abdominis

Triceps brachii

Internal obliques (deep)

External obliques

Hip flexors (deep)

Pelvic floor (hidden)

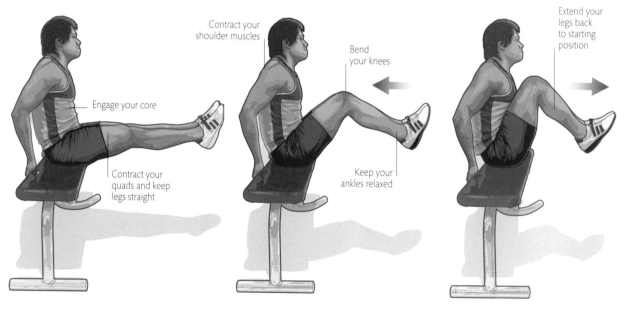

Engage your core

Contract your quads and keep legs straight

Contract your shoulder muscles

Bend your knees

Keep your ankles relaxed

Extend your legs back to starting position

1 Sit on the bench, supporting yourself by gripping the pad behind you. Lift your legs together, keeping your toes pointed.

2 Keeping your legs and feet together, bend the knees and bring them towards your chest. Pull your torso forwards a little for balance.

3 Bring your knees as close to your chest as possible. Reverse the sequence to return to the start position, slowly and with control.

V SIT-UP

TARGET MUSCLES	TARGET MOVEMENT
■ Rectus abdominis	
■ Transverse abdominis	
■ Pelvic floor	
■ Hip flexors	

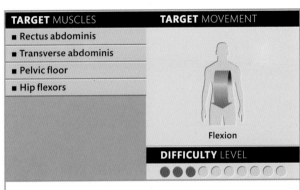

Flexion

DIFFICULTY LEVEL

A similar movement to the V leg-raise (**opposite**), this exercise requires greater core stability to perform as you do not have the support of the bench. Good form is crucial. Control the movement with your abdominals and keep your neck and shoulders relaxed.

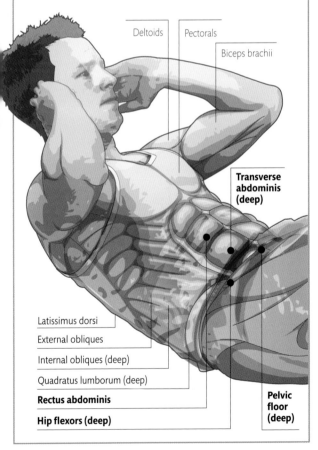

Deltoids

Pectorals

Biceps brachii

Transverse abdominis (deep)

Latissimus dorsi

External obliques

Internal obliques (deep)

Quadratus lumborum (deep)

Rectus abdominis

Hip flexors (deep)

Pelvic floor (deep)

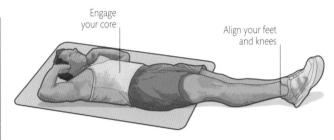

Engage your core

Align your feet and knees

1 Lie with your feet together and your hands touching the sides of your head. Engage the core, and raise your head and feet slightly off the floor.

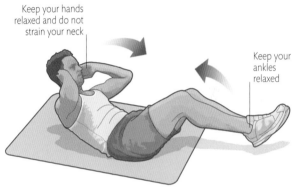

Keep your hands relaxed and do not strain your neck

Keep your ankles relaxed

2 Keeping your feet and knees together, simultaneously crunch up with your upper body as you bend your knees and bring them towards your chest. Control the movement with your core.

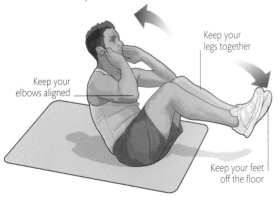

Keep your legs together

Keep your elbows aligned

Keep your feet off the floor

3 Continue the crunching movement, bringing your knees and chest towards each other as far as you can. Return by extending your hips and knees and leaning back to counterbalance. Repeat as required.

SWIM

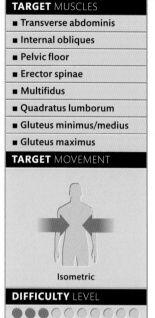

TARGET MUSCLES

- Transverse abdominis
- Internal obliques
- Pelvic floor
- Erector spinae
- Multifidus
- Quadratus lumborum
- Gluteus minimus/medius
- Gluteus maximus

TARGET MOVEMENT

Isometric

DIFFICULTY LEVEL

This exercise works the stabilizing muscles on either side of your spine, along with your buttocks and hamstrings. When performing it, try to make the movements on each side as symmetrical and balanced as possible. As you progress, you can speed the exercise up.

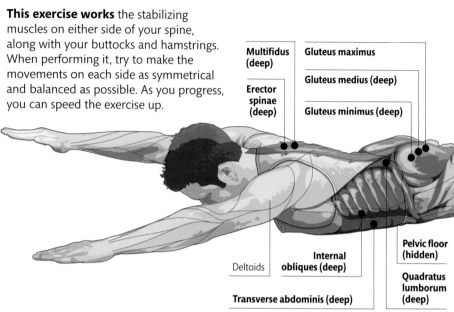

Multifidus (deep)

Gluteus maximus

Gluteus medius (deep)

Erector spinae (deep)

Gluteus minimus (deep)

Pelvic floor (hidden)

Quadratus lumborum (deep)

Deltoids

Internal obliques (deep)

Transverse abdominis (deep)

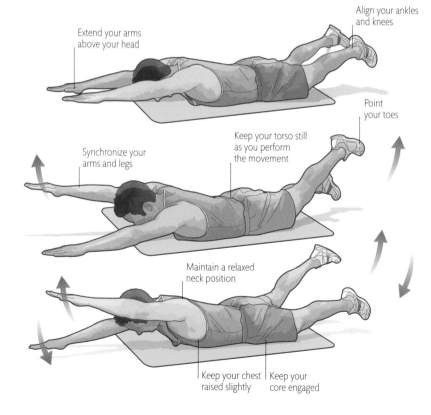

1 Lie face down on the floor, with your arms extended above your head, palms downwards. Engaging your core, raise your arms and legs slightly off the floor and stretch your neck to elongate your torso.

Extend your arms above your head

Align your ankles and knees

Point your toes

2 Lift your right arm and left leg at the same time, keeping all your limbs as straight as possible. Control the movement with your core to avoid rotating your torso and "cheating" the movement.

Synchronize your arms and legs

Keep your torso still as you perform the movement

3 Simultaneously lower your right arm and left leg, and lift your left arm and right leg. Alternate for the required number of repetitions.

Maintain a relaxed neck position

Keep your chest raised slightly

Keep your core engaged

SUPER-SLOW BICYCLE

TARGET MUSCLES

- Rectus abdominis
- Transverse abdominis
- External obliques
- Internal obliques
- Pelvic floor
- Multifidus
- Quadratus lumborum

TARGET MOVEMENT

Rotation

DIFFICULTY LEVEL

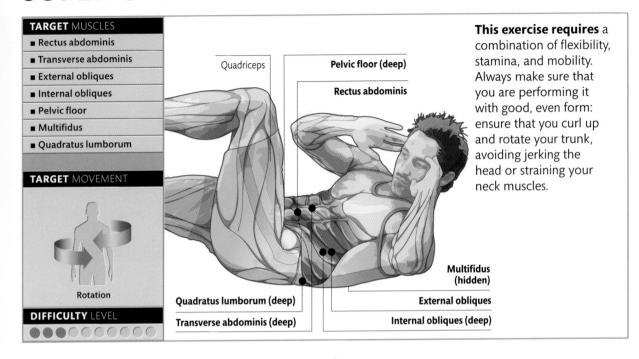

Quadriceps

Pelvic floor (deep)

Rectus abdominis

Multifidus (hidden)

External obliques

Internal obliques (deep)

Quadratus lumborum (deep)

Transverse abdominis (deep)

This exercise requires a combination of flexibility, stamina, and mobility. Always make sure that you are performing it with good, even form: ensure that you curl up and rotate your trunk, avoiding jerking the head or straining your neck muscles.

1 Lie on your back with your pelvis in a neutral position, and your knees and hips bent at a right angle. Place your hands on your temples.

2 Using your core to control the movement, slowly bring your left elbow and right knee together, rotating your torso to the right and extending your left leg.

3 Switch sides, bringing your right elbow towards the left knee and extending your right leg. Repeat the sequence for the desired number of repetitions.

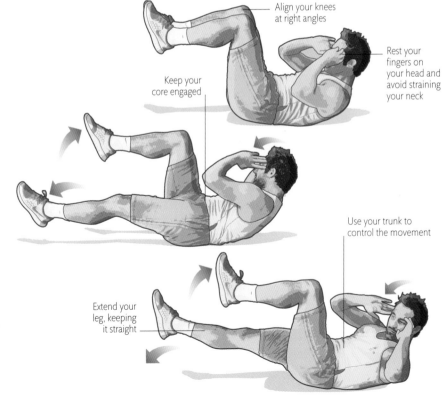

Align your knees at right angles

Rest your fingers on your head and avoid straining your neck

Keep your core engaged

Use your trunk to control the movement

Extend your leg, keeping it straight

SPRINTER SIT-UP

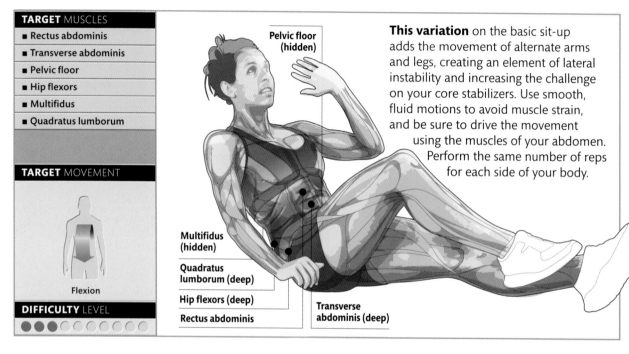

TARGET MUSCLES

- Rectus abdominis
- Transverse abdominis
- Pelvic floor
- Hip flexors
- Multifidus
- Quadratus lumborum

TARGET MOVEMENT

Flexion

DIFFICULTY LEVEL

Pelvic floor (hidden)

Multifidus (hidden)

Quadratus lumborum (deep)

Hip flexors (deep)

Rectus abdominis

Transverse abdominis (deep)

This variation on the basic sit-up adds the movement of alternate arms and legs, creating an element of lateral instability and increasing the challenge on your core stabilizers. Use smooth, fluid motions to avoid muscle strain, and be sure to drive the movement using the muscles of your abdomen. Perform the same number of reps for each side of your body.

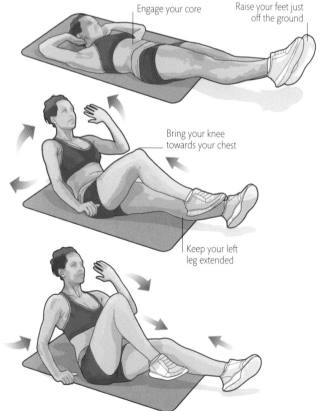

1 Lie on your back with your hands touching the sides of the head and your elbows back and aligned. Stretch your legs and raise your head and feet just off the ground.

Engage your core

Raise your feet just off the ground

2 Crunch up with your abs and bring your right knee towards your chest. At the same time, extend your left elbow out in front of you and drop your right arm to your side.

Bring your knee towards your chest

Keep your left leg extended

3 Extend the movement further until you assume a similar position to that of a runner, with your right knee and left elbow roughly aligned. Slowly return to the start position and switch sides.

HORIZONTAL BALANCE

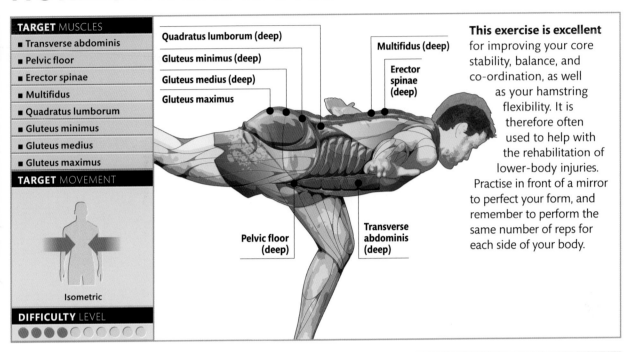

TARGET MUSCLES
- Transverse abdominis
- Pelvic floor
- Erector spinae
- Multifidus
- Quadratus lumborum
- Gluteus minimus
- Gluteus medius
- Gluteus maximus

TARGET MOVEMENT

Isometric

DIFFICULTY LEVEL

Quadratus lumborum (deep)
Gluteus minimus (deep)
Gluteus medius (deep)
Gluteus maximus
Multifidus (deep)
Erector spinae (deep)
Pelvic floor (deep)
Transverse abdominis (deep)

This exercise is excellent for improving your core stability, balance, and co-ordination, as well as your hamstring flexibility. It is therefore often used to help with the rehabilitation of lower-body injuries. Practise in front of a mirror to perfect your form, and remember to perform the same number of reps for each side of your body.

PROGRESSION

Performing the exercise on a half-exercise ball makes for a much more challenging version of the movement. Maintain good form and perform the same number of repetitions for each side.

Keep your leg in line with your back

Keep your spine straight and aligned

Keep your core engaged

Bend your left knee to a maximum of 20–30 degrees

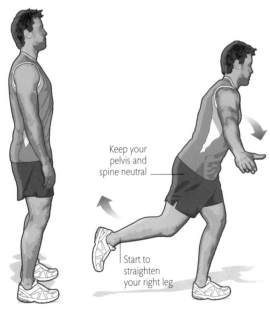

Keep your pelvis and spine neutral

Start to straighten your right leg

1 Stand upright with your shoulder and hips aligned, and your back in a neutral position, and your feet shoulder-width apart.

2 Bend forwards at your hips, lifting your right leg back and transferring the weight on to your left leg, bending your knee slightly, and lifting your arms as you do so.

3 Continue until your body is as close as you can get to parallel with the floor. Hold, then reverse the movement slowly and with control. Repeat as required and switch sides.

BRIDGE

TARGET MUSCLES	TARGET MOVEMENT
■ Rectus abdominis	
■ Transverse abdominis	
■ Pelvic floor	
■ Erector spinae	
■ Multifidus	
■ Quadratus lumborum	
■ Gluteus minimus	
■ Gluteus medius	Isometric
■ Gluteus maximus	DIFFICULTY LEVEL

This simple but effective exercise activates the stabilizing muscles of your lower back and buttocks, and offers additional benefits to your hamstrings. It is an important core-stabilizing movement for helping to improve your posture – especially if you spend a lot of time sitting at a desk. It is a very versatile exercise with a wide range of potential variations and progressions.

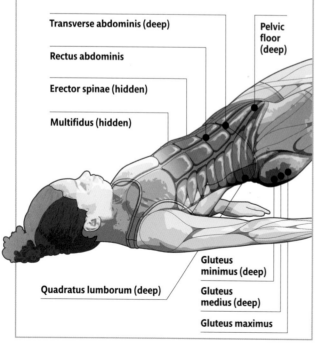

Transverse abdominis (deep)

Rectus abdominis

Erector spinae (hidden)

Multifidus (hidden)

Pelvic floor (deep)

Quadratus lumborum (deep)

Gluteus minimus (deep)

Gluteus medius (deep)

Gluteus maximus

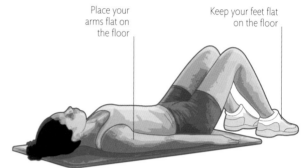

Place your arms flat on the floor

Keep your feet flat on the floor

1 Lie on your back with your knees bent and your feet flat on the floor, hip-width apart. Keep your arms at your sides, palms facing down. Relax your head and shoulders.

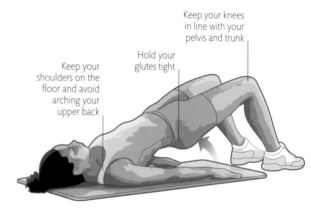

Keep your knees in line with your pelvis and trunk

Hold your glutes tight

Keep your shoulders on the floor and avoid arching your upper back

2 Engaging your core, slowly lift your buttocks off the floor until the body is in a straight line from your knees to your shoulders.

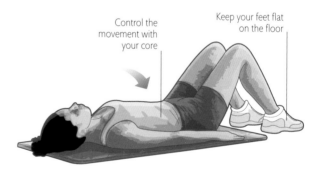

Control the movement with your core

Keep your feet flat on the floor

3 Hold at the top of the movement, then reverse slowly and with control to return to the starting position.

PROGRESSION 1

A development of the basic bridge, this version of the exercise is performed on one leg and so introduces an element of instability, forcing you to control the rotation and tilt of your pelvis.

This puts more stress on your deep abdominals and lower back muscles. It is important to ensure that you keep your hips level and your spine aligned throughout the movement.

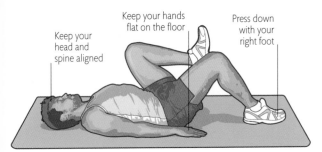

Keep your head and spine aligned

Keep your hands flat on the floor

Press down with your right foot

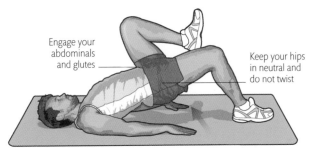

Engage your abdominals and glutes

Keep your hips in neutral and do not twist

1 Lie with your knees bent and your legs hip-width apart. Keeping your right foot on the floor, raise your left knee up and hold it above your hip, ensuring you maintain hip alignment before you begin.

2 Lift your buttocks as high as you can without dropping one side, ensuring you maintain neutral hip position. Hold briefly, then reverse to return to the start position and switch legs.

PROGRESSION 2

Placing a stability disc beneath your upper back and placing your arms across your chest removes the main support, meaning that your core has to work harder to keep you stable and balanced. Lie on your back with your knees bent at right angles and your feet flat on the floor, hip-width apart. Cross your arms over your chest, and slowly lift your buttocks until your body is in the bridge position. Hold and return to the start position.

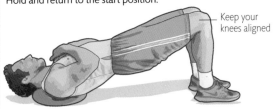

Keep your knees aligned

PROGRESSION 3

Assuming the bridge position with your feet placed in bodyweight suspension bands adds a challenging element of instability that requires even greater core strength and stability to control. Carry out the movement in this progression as normal, ensuring you maintain good form.

Maintain a straight line from your shoulders to knees

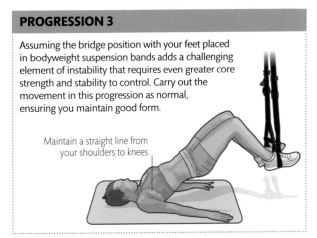

PROGRESSION 4

Performing the one-legged bridge on a half-exercise ball further increases the instability of the position. Lie with your arms at your sides. With your feet on the ball and the weight on your upper back and arms, raise your buttocks. Straighten one leg in line with your back. Hold, then relax and switch your legs.

Engage your core

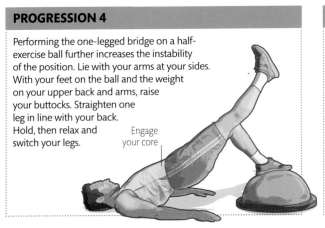

PROGRESSION 5

The multi-directional instability of an exercise ball means this version of the movement requires great core control and balance. Lie on your back and plant your feet on the ball. Supporting the weight with your upper back and arms, raise your buttocks. Hold, then return to the start position.

Position your feet on the exercise ball

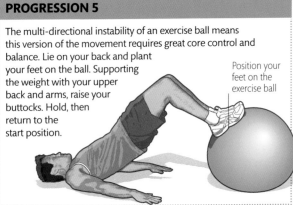

DOUBLE-LEG LOWER AND LIFT

TARGET MUSCLES
- Rectus abdominis
- Transverse abdominis
- Pelvic floor
- Hip flexors
- Multifidus
- Quadratus lumborum
- Gluteus minimus
- Gluteus medius

TARGET MOVEMENT

Isometric

DIFFICULTY LEVEL

This reasonably demanding core exercise helps build stability in the deep core muscles of your spine as well as providing a great workout for your abs. Make sure that you maintain good form throughout to avoid placing any stress on your lower back.

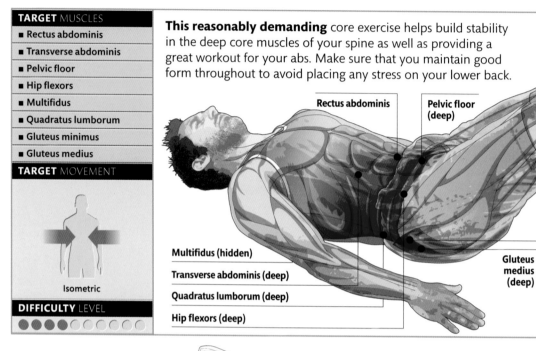

Rectus abdominis

Pelvic floor (deep)

Multifidus (hidden)

Transverse abdominis (deep)

Quadratus lumborum (deep)

Hip flexors (deep)

Gluteus medius (deep)

Gluteus minimus (deep)

1 Lie on your back with your arms placed by your sides. Raise your legs into a vertical position, keeping your knees and feet together and your back and hips neutral.

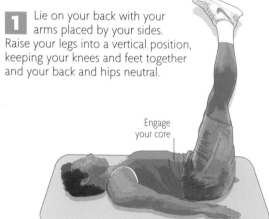

Engage your core

2 Slowly lower your legs, keeping your feet and knees together, controlling the movement with your core and keeping your torso stationary.

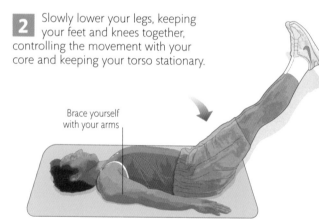

Brace yourself with your arms

3 Continue the movement until your feet are as near to the floor as you can get, maintaining a neutral back. Hold this position briefly, then slowly lift your legs back to the start position, with a controlled, smooth motion. Avoid lifting your lower back as you repeat.

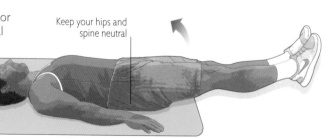

Keep your hips and spine neutral

VARIATION

This version of the exercise works each of your legs in turn, introducing an element of lateral instability. Focus on good, even form in your movements.

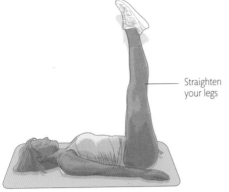

Straighten your legs

1 Lie on your back with your palms facing down and your legs raised vertically.

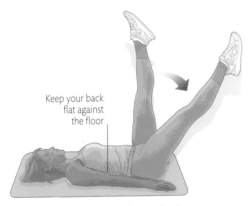

Keep your back flat against the floor

2 Keeping your left leg held upright, lower your right leg slowly and under control.

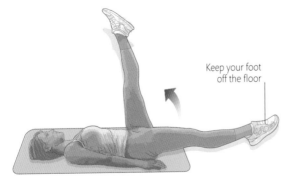

Keep your foot off the floor

3 Pause with your right leg as low as you can get, without lifting your back, then return to the start position. Alternate your legs throughout the exercise.

PROGRESSION 1

Holding an exercise ball between your feet as you perform the movement increases its intensity, making your core muscles work harder, while also recruiting additional muscles in your inner thighs. Grasp the exercise ball with the inside of your feet and raise your legs into a vertical position. Lower the ball to a few centimetres above the floor, hold briefly and return to the start position.

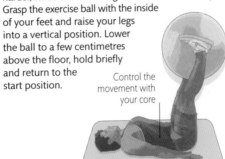

Control the movement with your core

PROGRESSION 2

To increase the intensity of the exercise further, carry it out with your shoulders off the floor in a held crunch position. This will help to further increase your core stamina, while removing the support of your upper back and shoulders. The position makes your core work much harder to keep you stable and balanced.

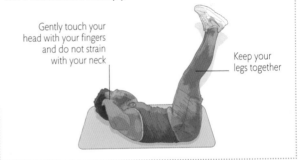

Gently touch your head with your fingers and do not strain with your neck

Keep your legs together

PROGRESSION 3

You can use the weight of a kettlebell to increase the load on the core and make the exercise even more challenging. Keeping your arms extended straight behind your head, hold the weight behind your head and a few centimetres off the floor as you lower your legs from a vertical position to a few inches off the floor.

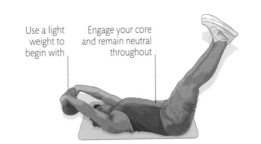

Use a light weight to begin with

Engage your core and remain neutral throughout

PLANK

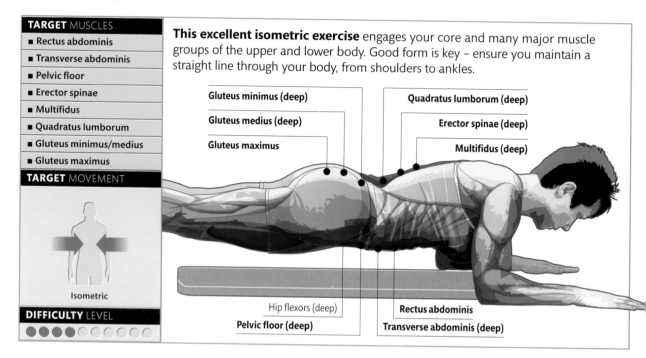

TARGET MUSCLES

- Rectus abdominis
- Transverse abdominis
- Pelvic floor
- Erector spinae
- Multifidus
- Quadratus lumborum
- Gluteus minimus/medius
- Gluteus maximus

TARGET MOVEMENT

Isometric

DIFFICULTY LEVEL

This excellent isometric exercise engages your core and many major muscle groups of the upper and lower body. Good form is key – ensure you maintain a straight line through your body, from shoulders to ankles.

Gluteus minimus (deep)

Gluteus medius (deep)

Gluteus maximus

Quadratus lumborum (deep)

Erector spinae (deep)

Multifidus (deep)

Hip flexors (deep)

Pelvic floor (deep)

Rectus abdominis

Transverse abdominis (deep)

1 Lie face down on an exercise mat with your elbows to your sides, your head facing forward, and palms flat on the floor.

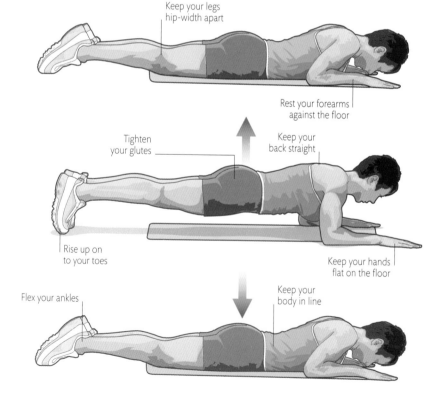

Keep your legs hip-width apart

Rest your forearms against the floor

Tighten your glutes

Keep your back straight

2 Engaging your core and glutes, raise your body from the floor, supporting your weight on your forearms and toes while breathing freely. Concentrate on maintaining a straight line through your core and legs.

Rise up on to your toes

Keep your hands flat on the floor

Flex your ankles

Keep your body in line

3 Hold the plank position, maintaining good form and keeping your glutes tensed, then return to the start position slowly and with good control.

PROGRESSION 1

Supporting your weight with only one arm and one leg introduces an element of instability, which your body has to brace itself against. Maintain a straight line through your raised arm and your raised leg, and be sure to repeat on both sides.

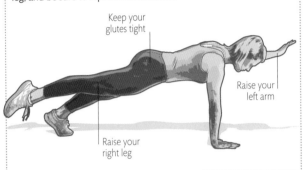

Keep your glutes tight

Raise your left arm

Raise your right leg

PROGRESSION 2

Placing your feet on a half-exercise ball adds a different kind of instability for your core muscles to work against. Begin by supporting your weight with your elbows on the floor, then raise yourself onto your hands.

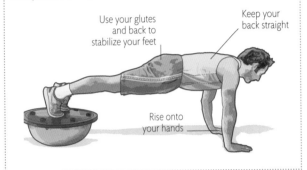

Use your glutes and back to stabilize your feet

Keep your back straight

Rise onto your hands

PROGRESSION 3

An exercise ball offers an even greater challenge than a half-exercise ball because it can move in all directions. As a result, this further adaptation of Progression 2 requires an even greater level of core stability to keep your body balanced. Begin by supporting your weight on your elbows, then raise yourself into position.

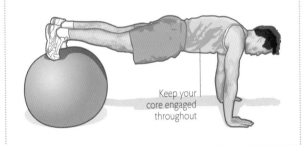

Keep your core engaged throughout

PROGRESSION 4

Once you have mastered the first three progressions you can make the plank even harder by raising your feet in bodyweight suspension straps. The straps make it even harder to stabilize your body, and so require excellent core stability and strength. Carry out the movement as normal with good control.

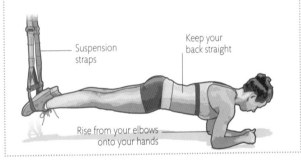

Suspension straps

Keep your back straight

Rise from your elbows onto your hands

PROGRESSION 5

This progression uses an exercise ball to generate instability in your upper body, which is harder to control with your core. Kneel with your feet slightly apart, and lean forwards to rest both hands on the ball before carefully raising your body up into a plank.

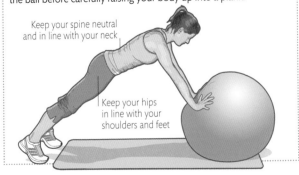

Keep your spine neutral and in line with your neck

Keep your hips in line with your shoulders and feet

PROGRESSION 6

Supporting your weight on the exercise ball with just one hand places a rotational force on your spinal muscles, making your core work even harder to stabilize your body. The position is potentially dangerous so do not attempt this before you have mastered the other progressions. Also, always balance the movement by repeating the plank on both sides.

Engage your core throughout

SIDE PLANK

TARGET MUSCLES	TARGET MOVEMENT
■ Transverse abdominis	
■ External obliques	
■ Internal obliques	
■ Pelvic floor	
■ Multifidus	
■ Quadratus lumborum	
■ Gluteus minimus	Isometric
■ Gluteus medius	**DIFFICULTY** LEVEL
■ Gluteus maximus	●●●●● ○○○○○

This excellent core exercise strengthens the stabilizing muscles of your spine, lower back, and glutes. While the basic position is relatively simple to achieve, maintaining good form is crucial to working your core in the right way. It is also important to ensure that you aim to hold the position for the same length of time on both sides of your body, in order to prevent imbalance.

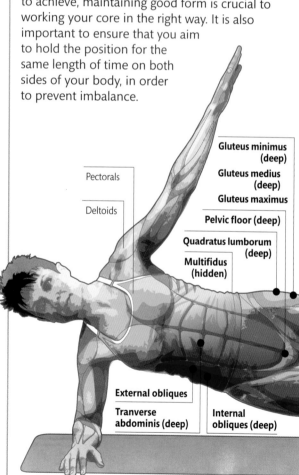

Pectorals

Deltoids

Gluteus minimus (deep)
Gluteus medius (deep)
Gluteus maximus
Pelvic floor (deep)
Quadratus lumborum (deep)
Multifidus (hidden)

External obliques
Tranverse abdominis (deep)
Internal obliques (deep)

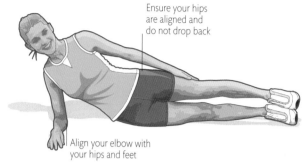

Ensure your hips are aligned and do not drop back

Align your elbow with your hips and feet

1 Lying on your right side, prop yourself up on your right forearm. Extend your legs and keep your feet together. Make sure that your right elbow is directly under your shoulder and in line with your hips. Rest your left arm along your side.

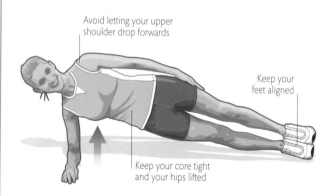

Avoid letting your upper shoulder drop forwards

Keep your feet aligned

Keep your core tight and your hips lifted

2 Engage the abdominals and push downwards through your right elbow to raise your hips off the ground, making sure that you keep the ribcage elevated and your shoulders in line with each other.

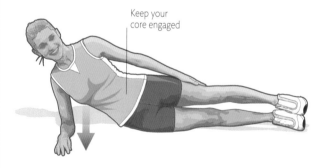

Keep your core engaged

3 Hold the position for eight seconds, then return to the start position for a further two seconds. Repeat as required, then switch sides.

PROGRESSION 1

This progression of the basic side plank adds an element of instability because of the raised arm. This makes your core work harder to keep your body stable and balanced.

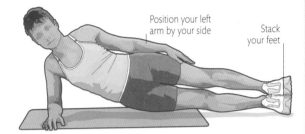

Position your left arm by your side

Stack your feet

1 Lie on your right side supported by your forearm, with your right elbow directly under your shoulder and in line with your hips, as in the original movement.

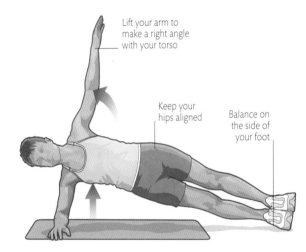

Lift your arm to make a right angle with your torso

Keep your hips aligned

Balance on the side of your foot

2 Raise your left arm until it is at a 90-degree angle to your torso, keeping your ribcage elevated and your shoulders aligned.

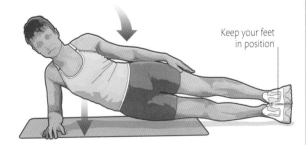

Keep your feet in position

3 Hold for eight seconds, and then return to the start position for two seconds. Repeat as required, before switching sides.

PROGRESSION 2

A development of Progression 1, this position involves raising both your free arm and leg, requiring even greater core stability and control to keep your body balanced.

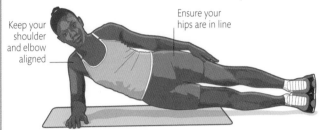

Keep your shoulder and elbow aligned

Ensure your hips are in line

1 Lying on your right side, prop yourself up on your right forearm. Extend your legs and keep your feet together. Position your supporting elbow under your shoulder and aligned with your hips. Rest your left arm on your side.

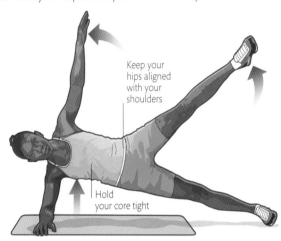

Keep your hips aligned with your shoulders

Hold your core tight

2 As you lift your hips into the plank position, raise your left arm and leg until you make a star shape, keeping your shoulders and hips aligned. Hold, then return to the start position. Repeat as required, then switch sides.

PROGRESSION 3

This further progression involves placing your feet in bodyweight suspension straps to increase the level of instability even further. Do not attempt this unless you have excellent core stability and strength.

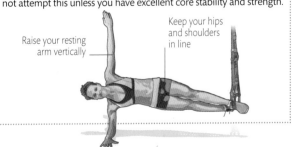

Raise your resting arm vertically

Keep your hips and shoulders in line

SINGLE-LEG EXTENSION AND STRETCH

TARGET MUSCLES	TARGET MOVEMENT
■ Rectus abdominis	
■ Transverse abdominis	
■ Internal obliques	
■ Pelvic floor	
■ Multifidus	
■ Quadratus lumborum	
■ Gluteus minimus	
■ Gluteus medius	Flexion

This core flexion movement is a good exercise for strengthening a number of your core muscles, and helps to improve your core stability and stamina, especially against lumbar extension and rotation.

DIFFICULTY LEVEL

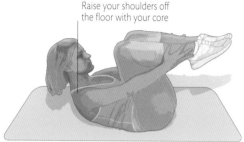

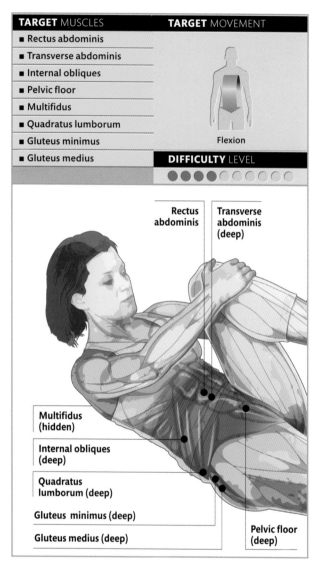

Rectus abdominis

Transverse abdominis (deep)

Multifidus (hidden)

Internal obliques (deep)

Quadratus lumborum (deep)

Gluteus minimus (deep)

Gluteus medius (deep)

Pelvic floor (deep)

Raise your shoulders off the floor with your core

1 Lying on your back, bring both knees over your hips and reach your hands to your shins. Lift your head and shoulders slightly off the floor, look towards your feet, and use your core to hold the position to avoid straining your neck.

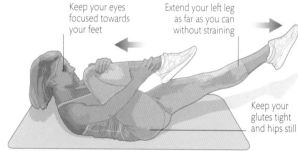

Keep your eyes focused towards your feet

Extend your left leg as far as you can without straining

Keep your glutes tight and hips still

2 Pull your right leg towards your body as you slowly extend your left leg out to 45 degrees. Keep your glutes and abdominals engaged to control the movement, and stay still and centred in your hips.

VARIATION

Performing the exercise with your head and shoulders resting on the floor helps ease possible strain on the neck and shoulders, while enabling a greater range of movement for your legs and hips. This would be a great place to start, before progressing and adding the curl up.

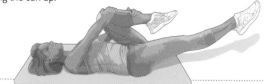

Maintain the curl in your back

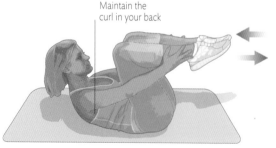

3 Return to the start position, maintaining your curl up and then switch to the other leg. Repeat as required.

DOUBLE-LEG EXTENSION AND STRETCH

TARGET MUSCLES

- Rectus abdominis
- Transverse abdominis
- Internal obliques
- Pelvic floor
- Multifidus
- Quadratus lumborum
- Gluteus minimus
- Gluteus medius

TARGET MOVEMENT

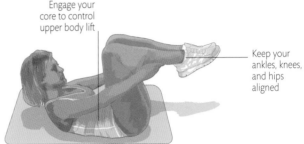

Flexion

DIFFICULTY LEVEL

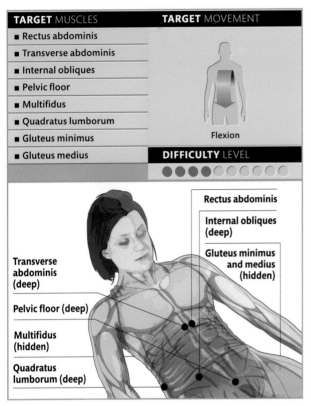

Rectus abdominis

Internal obliques (deep)

Gluteus minimus and medius (hidden)

Transverse abdominis (deep)

Pelvic floor (deep)

Multifidus (hidden)

Quadratus lumborum (deep)

VARIATION

If you are concerned about placing strain on the neck to begin with, try a variation of the exercise with your head resting flat on the floor. Extend your legs and arms outwards at the same angle, then return to the start position.

PROGRESSION

Once you have mastered the basic exercise, try as before but now extending your arms above your head at the same time as stretching your legs outwards to increase the level of instability. Keep your head off the floor and then return to the start position.

This exercise works in a similar way to the single-leg extension and stretch (opposite), but adds load on your lower abs. Ensure that your neck and shoulders are relaxed throughout to avoid straining.

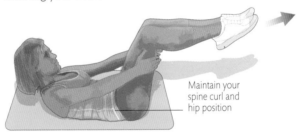

Engage your core to control upper body lift

Keep your ankles, knees, and hips aligned

1 Lying on your back, bring both knees over your hips and reach your hands to your shins. Lift your head and shoulders slightly off the floor, look towards your feet, and use your core to hold the position to avoid straining your neck.

Maintain your spine curl and hip position

2 Holding your core and glutes tight, extend your legs forwards with control, without tilting your hips. Keep your head and shoulders raised slightly and your neck relaxed.

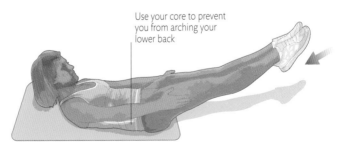

Use your core to prevent you from arching your lower back

3 Fully straighten your legs without letting your back arch off the floor, keeping your core engaged and your head raised. Hold briefly, then return to the start.

INTERMEDIATE

The exercises in this section build on those in Foundation, with the challenges of added instability, movement, weight, and power to make your core work harder and with greater functionality. Concentration and good technique are vital, and it is important that you can perform the less-advanced exercises with confidence before you try any of these.

PARTNER BALL SWAP

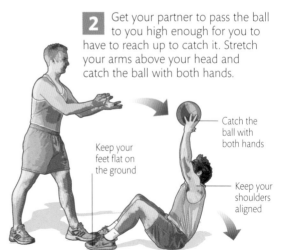

TARGET MUSCLES
- Rectus abdominis
- Transverse abdominis
- Internal obliques
- Pelvic floor
- Hip flexors

TARGET MOVEMENT

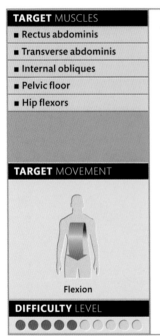

Flexion

DIFFICULTY LEVEL

A development of the basic sit-up, this exercise introduces a more powerful, dynamic movement with the weight of a medicine ball. It provides an excellent workout for your abdominals with additional benefits to your shoulders, chest, and arms. You will need the help of a willing partner to assist with throwing and catching the ball.

Internal obliques (deep)

Transverse abdominis (deep)

Rectus abdominis

Pelvic floor (deep)

Hip flexors (deep)

1 Sit up straight on the floor with your core engaged, your legs bent at right angles, and your feet flat. Get your partner to stand by your feet, holding a medicine ball.

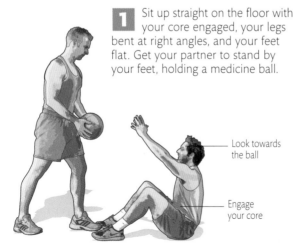

Look towards the ball

Engage your core

2 Get your partner to pass the ball to you high enough for you to have to reach up to catch it. Stretch your arms above your head and catch the ball with both hands.

Keep your feet flat on the ground

Catch the ball with both hands

Keep your shoulders aligned

3 Using the momentum of the ball, but controlling the movement with your core, roll your upper body backwards until your back reaches the floor. Extend your arms above your head as you do so.

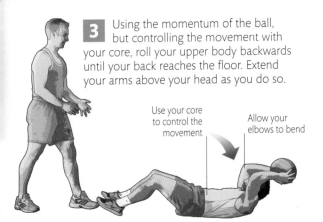

Use your core to control the movement

Allow your elbows to bend

4 Keeping your elbows bent, continue extending your arms until the ball touches the ground.

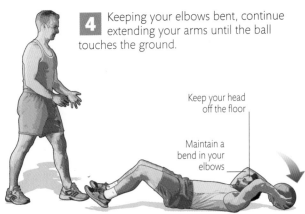

Keep your head off the floor

Maintain a bend in your elbows

5 Pause briefly in this position, then use your core (and not the momentum of your arms) to raise your upper body into a sit-up with a smooth, dynamic movement.

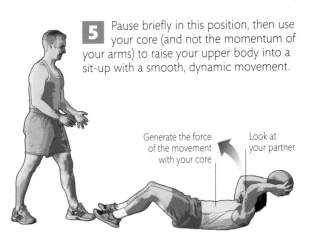

Generate the force of the movement with your core

Look at your partner

6 Continue the dynamic movement of the sit-up, raising the ball held above your head as you do so.

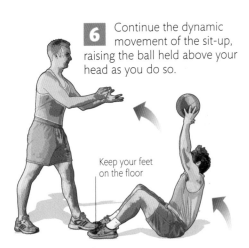

Keep your feet on the floor

7 Release the ball to your partner as you reach an upright position, using only the force generated by the movement from your core. Do not try to throw it.

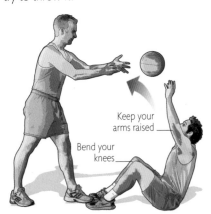

Keep your arms raised

Bend your knees

8 Continue the movement to the start position, with your knees bent and arms outstretched as your partner catches the ball.

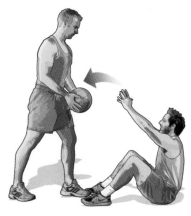

PROGRESSION

Varying the position in which you catch the ball makes the exercise more challenging and introduces an element of rotational instability that recruits a number of additional core muscles. Repeat the same sequence as the main exercise, asking your partner to vary the position and angle of the throw to balance the workout across your core.

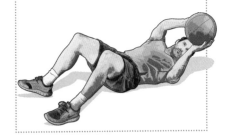

HANGING KNEE-UP

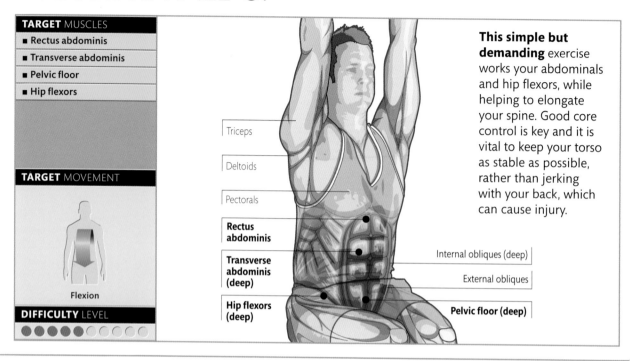

TARGET MUSCLES
- Rectus abdominis
- Transverse abdominis
- Pelvic floor
- Hip flexors

TARGET MOVEMENT

Flexion

DIFFICULTY LEVEL

Triceps

Deltoids

Pectorals

Rectus abdominis

Transverse abdominis (deep)

Hip flexors (deep)

Internal obliques (deep)

External obliques

Pelvic floor (deep)

This simple but demanding exercise works your abdominals and hip flexors, while helping to elongate your spine. Good core control is key and it is vital to keep your torso as stable as possible, rather than jerking with your back, which can cause injury.

WINDMILL

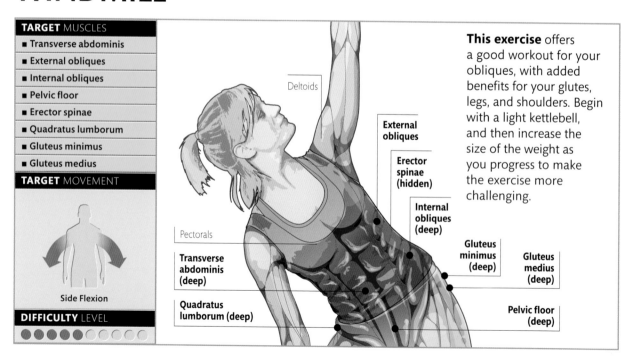

TARGET MUSCLES
- Transverse abdominis
- External obliques
- Internal obliques
- Pelvic floor
- Erector spinae
- Quadratus lumborum
- Gluteus minimus
- Gluteus medius

TARGET MOVEMENT

Side Flexion

DIFFICULTY LEVEL

Deltoids

External obliques

Erector spinae (hidden)

Internal obliques (deep)

Gluteus minimus (deep)

Gluteus medius (deep)

Pectorals

Transverse abdominis (deep)

Quadratus lumborum (deep)

Pelvic floor (deep)

This exercise offers a good workout for your obliques, with added benefits for your glutes, legs, and shoulders. Begin with a light kettlebell, and then increase the size of the weight as you progress to make the exercise more challenging.

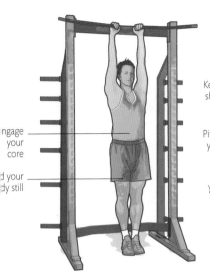

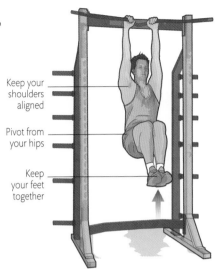

ngage
your
core

d your
dy still

Keep your
shoulders
aligned

Pivot from
your hips

Keep
your feet
together

1 Hang from a stable chin-up bar using an overhand grip with your arms straight and shoulder-width apart. Keeping your body as still as possible and your legs together, engage your core.

2 Keeping your body still and your legs together, raise your knees upwards, using your core to control the movement, until your hips and knees are at right angles. Pause, then return to the start position with good control.

PROGRESSION

Once you have mastered the basic exercise, you can increase the load on your core by lifting each leg alternately. Assume the same start position and raise your left leg as high as you can, keeping it straight and controlling the movement with your core. Hold briefly, then return to the start position and repeat with your right leg.

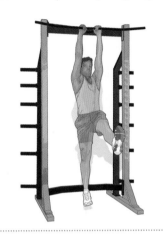

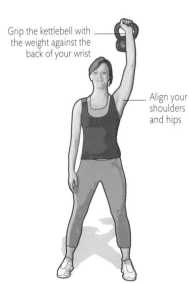

Grip the kettlebell with
the weight against the
back of your wrist

Align your
shoulders
and hips

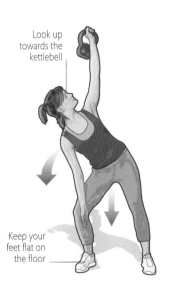

Look up
towards the
kettlebell

Keep your
feet flat on
the floor

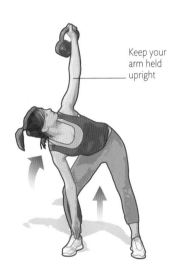

Keep your
arm held
upright

1 Stand with your feet slightly more than shoulder-width apart, holding a kettlebell in your left hand. Raise the weight above your left shoulder, allowing your right arm to hang by your side.

2 Keeping the kettlebell aloft and pivoting at your hips, drop your torso to the right, reaching towards the floor with your right arm and bending your right knee. Turn your head in the direction of the kettlebell as you do so.

3 Continue reaching down as far as you can with your right hand, keeping the kettlebell in position and your head turned towards it. Hold briefly, then return to the start position. Complete your reps, then switch sides.

GOOD MORNING

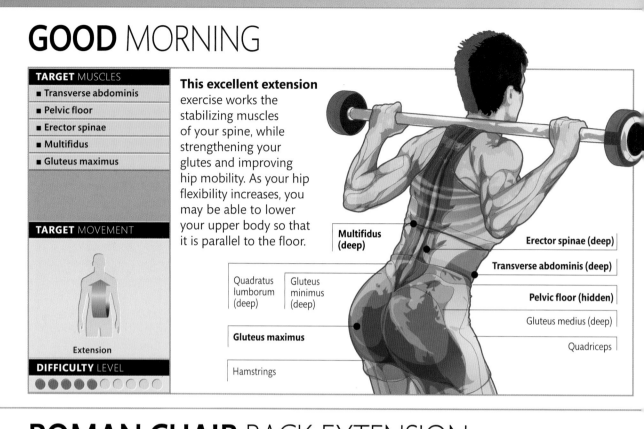

TARGET MUSCLES

- Transverse abdominis
- Pelvic floor
- Erector spinae
- Multifidus
- Gluteus maximus

TARGET MOVEMENT

Extension

DIFFICULTY LEVEL

This excellent extension exercise works the stabilizing muscles of your spine, while strengthening your glutes and improving hip mobility. As your hip flexibility increases, you may be able to lower your upper body so that it is parallel to the floor.

Multifidus (deep)

Erector spinae (deep)

Transverse abdominis (deep)

Quadratus lumborum (deep)

Gluteus minimus (deep)

Pelvic floor (hidden)

Gluteus medius (deep)

Gluteus maximus

Quadriceps

Hamstrings

ROMAN CHAIR BACK EXTENSION

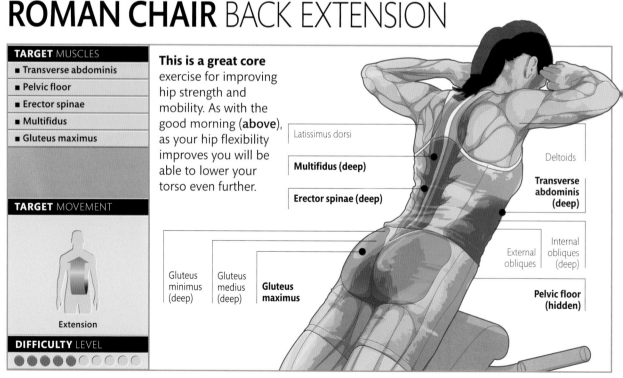

TARGET MUSCLES

- Transverse abdominis
- Pelvic floor
- Erector spinae
- Multifidus
- Gluteus maximus

TARGET MOVEMENT

Extension

DIFFICULTY LEVEL

This is a great core exercise for improving hip strength and mobility. As with the good morning (**above**), as your hip flexibility improves you will be able to lower your torso even further.

Latissimus dorsi

Deltoids

Multifidus (deep)

Erector spinae (deep)

Transverse abdominis (deep)

Gluteus minimus (deep)

Gluteus medius (deep)

Gluteus maximus

External obliques

Internal obliques (deep)

Pelvic floor (hidden)

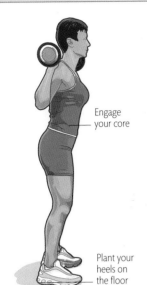
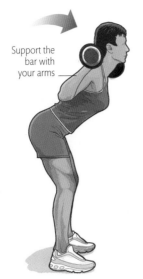
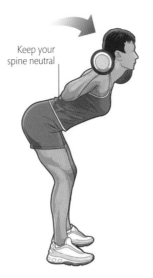
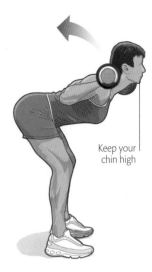

Engage your core

Plant your heels on the floor

Support the bar with your arms

Keep your spine neutral

Keep your chin high

1 Holding your body upright, position a barbell behind your neck and resting on the upper back. Keep your knees slightly bent and your spine neutral.

2 Bending slightly at your knees and hips, start to lean forwards under control. Keep your chin up – it will stop you from rounding your back.

3 Lean forwards by pivoting at your hip. Continue lowering your chest, keeping your back neutral and allowing your knees to bend slightly.

4 Flex as far as you can. With practice, your back may be parallel to the floor. Return to the start position, breathing out as you go.

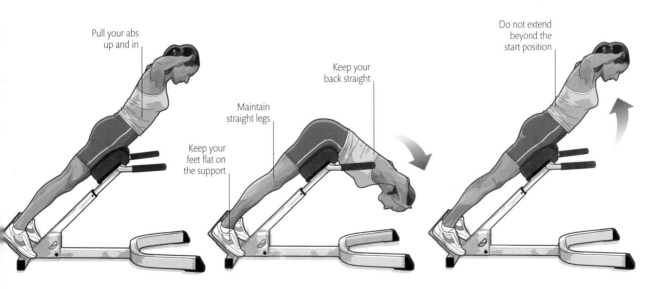

Pull your abs up and in

Keep your feet flat on the support

Maintain straight legs

Keep your back straight

Do not extend beyond the start position

1 Position your thighs on the pads of the Roman chair so that your hips are free to flex. Your feet should be flat on the foot supports, your spine neutral, and your elbows pointing out.

2 Flex at your hips and drop your upper body towards the floor, keeping your back flat. Stop bending when the flexibility of your hamstrings restricts further movement.

3 Return to the start position, contracting your hamstrings, glutes, and spinal erectors. Do not extend beyond the start position as you may injure your back.

O-BAR ROTATION

TARGET MUSCLES

- Transverse abdominis
- External obliques
- Internal obliques
- Pelvic floor
- Quadratus lumborum
- Gluteus minimus
- Gluteus medius

TARGET MOVEMENT

Rotation

DIFFICULTY LEVEL

This excellent rotational exercise uses an arcing movement that works a large group of muscles in unison. As a result it offers a useful full-body multi-joint movement that makes a good addition to any core-strength exercise programme.

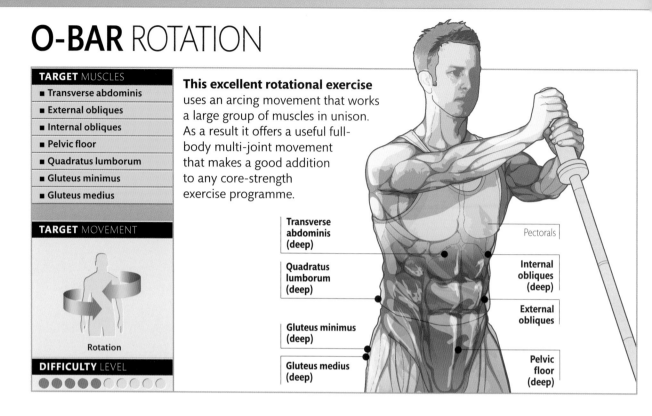

Transverse abdominis (deep)

Pectorals

Quadratus lumborum (deep)

Internal obliques (deep)

External obliques

Gluteus minimus (deep)

Gluteus medius (deep)

Pelvic floor (deep)

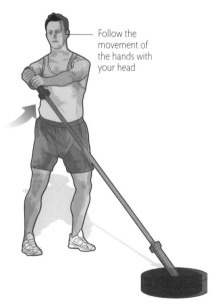

Follow the movement of the hands with your head

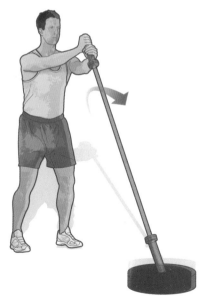

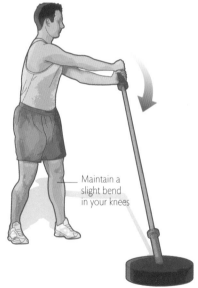

Maintain a slight bend in your knees

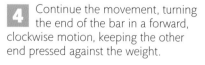

4 Continue the movement, turning the end of the bar in a forward, clockwise motion, keeping the other end pressed against the weight.

5 Follow the movement back and through the start position to your left, keeping your core engaged and maintaining good form.

6 Control the movement to your left, keeping your legs still and moving from your hip, and pivoting the bar from the weight on the floor.

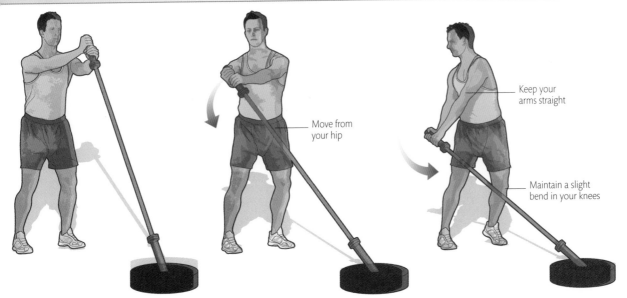

1 Position a heavy weight disc on the floor in front of you, and place one end of an Olympic bar in its centre. Grip the end of the bar with both hands and angle it towards you. Stand with your feet slightly wider than shoulder-width apart.

2 Keeping your feet, knees, and hips aligned, rotate the bar across your body to your right, maintaining straight arms, and controlling the movement by engaging your core and pivoting from your hips.

Move from your hip

3 Continuing the movement to your right, rotate the bar all the way around to waist level on your right-hand side, following it with your shoulders and head. Keep your arms straight throughout the movement.

Keep your arms straight

Maintain a slight bend in your knees

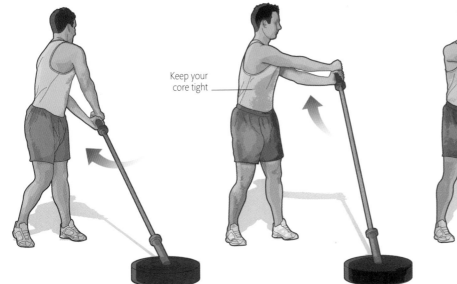

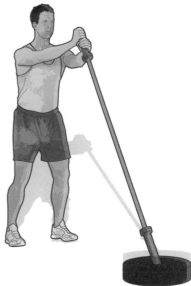

Keep your core tight

7 Control the motion of the bar all the way to waist level on your left, twisting at your hip at the edge of the movement.

8 Bring the bar back towards the start position in an anti-clockwise arc, straightening your legs and keeping your core engaged.

9 Complete the arc of movement to return to the start position, maintaining good form. Repeat the sequence as required and relax.

STANDING PLATE TWIST

TARGET MUSCLES	TARGET MOVEMENT
■ Transverse abdominis	
■ External obliques	
■ Internal obliques	
■ Pelvic floor	
■ Erector spinae	
■ Multifidus	
■ Quadratus lumborum	Rotation

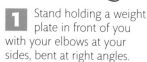

DIFFICULTY LEVEL

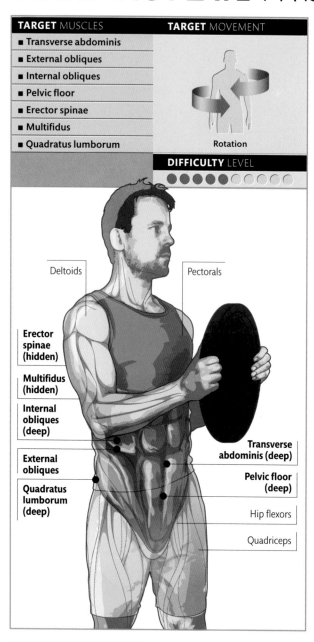

Deltoids

Pectorals

Erector spinae (hidden)

Multifidus (hidden)

Internal obliques (deep)

External obliques

Quadratus lumborum (deep)

Transverse abdominis (deep)

Pelvic floor (deep)

Hip flexors

Quadriceps

WARNING!

Ensure that you hold the weight plate close to your torso with your elbows at 90 degrees. If the plate is held away from your body this will place unwanted stress on the shoulders and lower back and could lead to potential injury.

This simple rotational exercise helps you to improve your spinal control, as you have to keep your hips stationary while you twist your upper body.

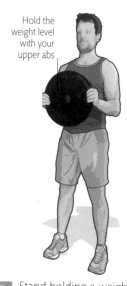

Hold the weight level with your upper abs

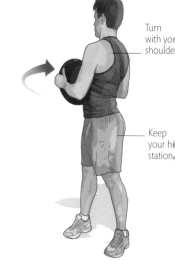

Turn with your shoulder

Keep your hips stationary

1 Stand holding a weight plate in front of you with your elbows at your sides, bent at right angles.

2 Slowly rotate your upper body to the right. Hold the position for a few seconds.

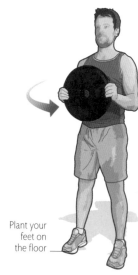

Plant your feet on the floor

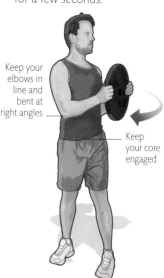

Keep your elbows in line and bent at right angles

Keep your core engaged

3 Slowly return to the start position, keeping your elbows at your sides and the weight the same distance from your upper abs.

4 Rotate through the start position to your left. Hold briefly, and repeat the exercise as required.

KETTLEBELL ROUND-BODY SWING

TARGET MUSCLES	TARGET MOVEMENT
■ Transverse abdominis	
■ Internal obliques	
■ Pelvic floor	
■ Erector spinae	
■ Multifidus	
■ Quadratus lumborum	

Isometric

DIFFICULTY LEVEL

This exercise provides a good workout for your core and upper body. Move slowly at first, only increasing speed once you have mastered the technique.

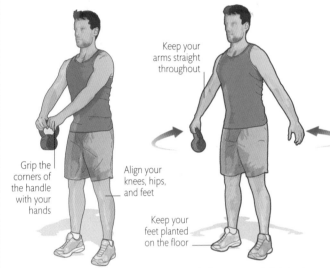

Keep your arms straight throughout

Grip the corners of the handle with your hands

Align your knees, hips, and feet

Keep your feet planted on the floor

1 Engaging your core, lift the kettlebell with both hands to hip height, keeping your arms straight.

2 Release your left hand, swing the weight to your right, and swing your left arm around to your left.

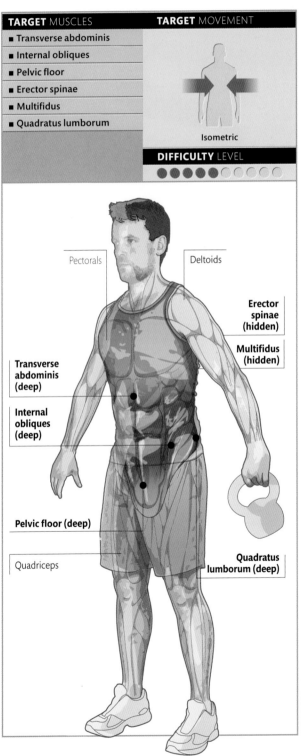

Pectorals

Deltoids

Erector spinae (hidden)

Multifidus (hidden)

Transverse abdominis (deep)

Internal obliques (deep)

Pelvic floor (deep)

Quadriceps

Quadratus lumborum (deep)

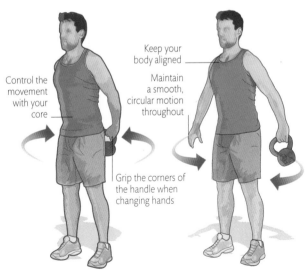

Control the movement with your core

Keep your body aligned

Maintain a smooth, circular motion throughout

Grip the corners of the handle when changing hands

3 In one smooth movement, swing your arms behind your lower back and pass the weight to your left hand.

4 With your left hand, bring the weight round to the start position. Repeat the movement as required, then switch direction.

MOUNTAIN CLIMBER

TARGET MUSCLES	TARGET MOVEMENT
■ Transverse abdominis	
■ Pelvic floor	
■ Hip flexors	
■ Erector spinae	
■ Multifidus	
■ Quadratus lumborum	
■ Gluteus medius	Isometric
■ Gluteus maximus	

DIFFICULTY LEVEL

The mountain climber is a dynamic movement that is excellent for building core stamina, while also improving your core strength, balance, and agility. It is especially useful if you have little equipment but want a challenging all-body workout.

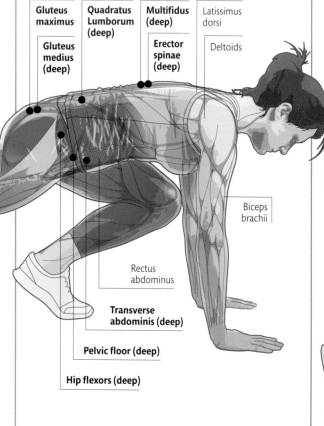

Gluteus maximus
Gluteus medius (deep)
Quadratus Lumborum (deep)
Multifidus (deep)
Erector spinae (deep)
Latissimus dorsi
Deltoids
Biceps brachii
Rectus abdominus
Transverse abdominis (deep)
Pelvic floor (deep)
Hip flexors (deep)

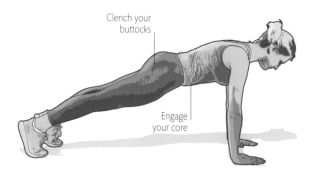

Clench your buttocks

Engage your core

1 Assume a normal press-up position with your weight on your hands and toes, your back and legs straight, and your hands shoulder-width apart.

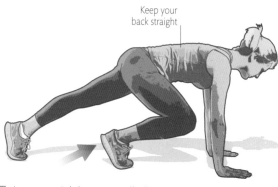

Keep your back straight

2 In one quick but controlled movement, bring your right knee up towards your chest, placing the ball of your right foot on the floor at the edge of the movement.

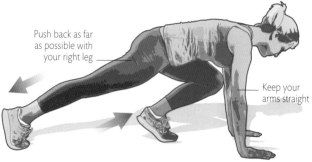

Push back as far as possible with your right leg

Keep your arms straight

3 Lightly spring up with your legs and switch feet, bringing your left foot up towards your chest as you push back with the right. Continue alternating your feet for the required number of reps, then relax to the start position.

RUSSIAN TWIST

TARGET MUSCLES

- Transverse abdominis
- External obliques
- Internal obliques
- Pelvic floor
- Erector spinae
- Multifidus
- Quadratus lumborum

TARGET MOVEMENT

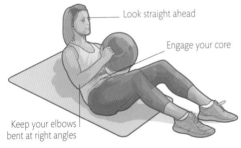

Rotation

DIFFICULTY LEVEL

This exercise is designed to improve your spinal flexibility, as well as building strength across your core. As with any movement that twists the spine, be sure to carry it out with good form and control.

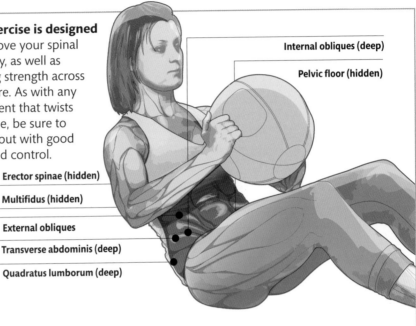

Internal obliques (deep)

Pelvic floor (hidden)

Erector spinae (hidden)

Multifidus (hidden)

External obliques

Transverse abdominis (deep)

Quadratus lumborum (deep)

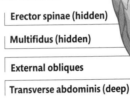

Look straight ahead

Engage your core

Keep your elbows bent at right angles

1 Sit with your knees slightly bent and your feet flat. Hold the ball out in front of you and lean back at a 45-degree angle, curving your torso slightly.

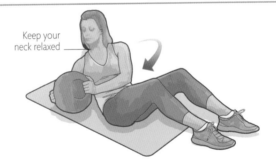

Keep your neck relaxed

2 Keeping your hips still, rotate your torso to your right as far as you can in a smooth motion, controlling the movement with your core, until the ball is close to the floor.

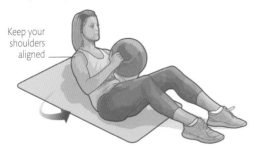

Keep your shoulders aligned

3 Hold briefly, then reverse back through to the start position, again controlling the movement from your core, and keeping your shoulders and hips relaxed.

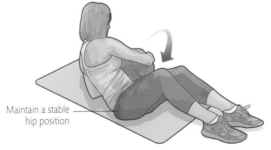

Maintain a stable hip position

4 Continue the movement to your left, rotating your torso and lowering the ball towards the floor. Hold for a few seconds, then return to the start position.

MEDICINE BALL SLAM

TARGET MUSCLES	**TARGET** MOVEMENT
■ Rectus abdominis	
■ Transverse abdominis	
■ Pelvic floor	

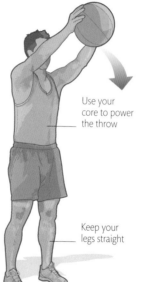

Flexion

DIFFICULTY LEVEL

This powerful, dynamic exercise offers your core a great workout, with added benefits for your shoulders. Focus on keeping your body as balanced as possible throughout, and start with a reasonably light ball, until you can carry out the movement with good form and confidence. You should enlist the help of a partner to retrieve the ball and prevent it from interfering with the activities of other gym users.

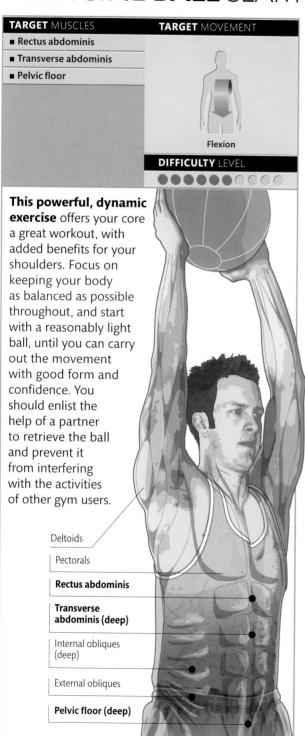

Deltoids

Pectorals

Rectus abdominis

Transverse abdominis (deep)

Internal obliques (deep)

External obliques

Pelvic floor (deep)

1 Holding a medicine ball in both hands, stand with both your feet shoulder-width apart and your back in a neutral position. Engaging your core, raise the medicine ball above your head, keeping your arms straight and your shoulders aligned with each other.

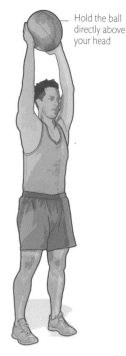

Hold the ball directly above your head

Use your core to power the throw

Keep your legs straight

2 In one powerful movement, drive the medicine ball down towards the floor in front of you, keeping your arms straight, pivoting at your shoulders, and driving the force with your core.

3 Release the ball at the bottom of the downwards movement, keeping your shoulders and hips aligned, and your legs straight. Ideally, you should drive the ball down hard enough to lift your body off the ground with the momentum generated by the movement. Retrieve the ball and repeat as required.

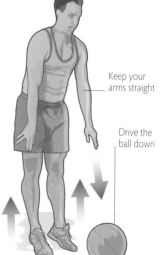

Keep your arms straight

Drive the ball down

MEDICINE BALL REVERSE THROW

TARGET MUSCLES	TARGET MOVEMENT
■ Transverse abdominis	
■ Pelvic floor	
■ Erector spinae	
■ Multifidus	
■ Gluteus maximus	

Extension

DIFFICULTY LEVEL

This excellent core extension exercise makes a good partner to the medicine ball slam (**opposite**). It is important to perfect your form with a lightweight ball to begin with. Also, you should always perform it with a partner, who can catch the ball for you and stop it interfering with other gym users.

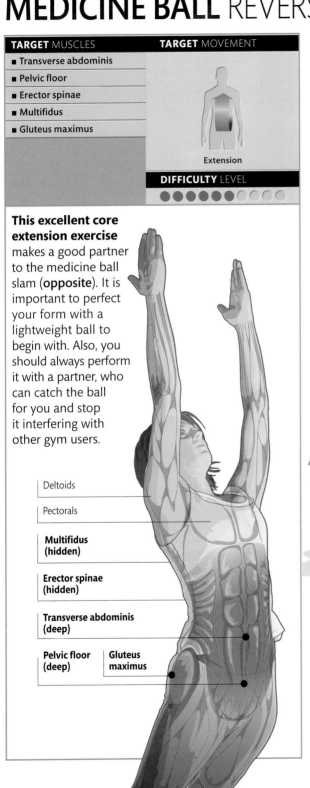

Deltoids

Pectorals

Multifidus (hidden)

Erector spinae (hidden)

Transverse abdominis (deep)

Pelvic floor (deep)

Gluteus maximus

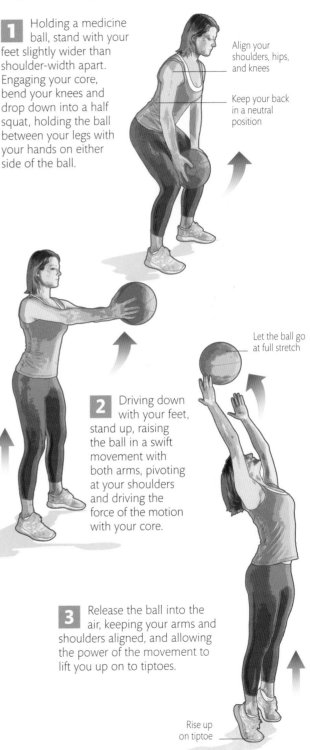

1 Holding a medicine ball, stand with your feet slightly wider than shoulder-width apart. Engaging your core, bend your knees and drop down into a half squat, holding the ball between your legs with your hands on either side of the ball.

Align your shoulders, hips, and knees

Keep your back in a neutral position

2 Driving down with your feet, stand up, raising the ball in a swift movement with both arms, pivoting at your shoulders and driving the force of the motion with your core.

Let the ball go at full stretch

3 Release the ball into the air, keeping your arms and shoulders aligned, and allowing the power of the movement to lift you up on to tiptoes.

Rise up on tiptoe

EXERCISE BALL BACK EXTENSION

TARGET MUSCLES	TARGET MOVEMENT
■ Transverse abdominis	
■ Pelvic floor	
■ Erector spinae	
■ Multifidus	
■ Quadratus lumborum	
■ Gluteus maximus	Extension

DIFFICULTY LEVEL

This exercise helps to balance your trunk by conditioning the stabilizing muscles of your lower back, challenging them against the movement of the exercise ball.

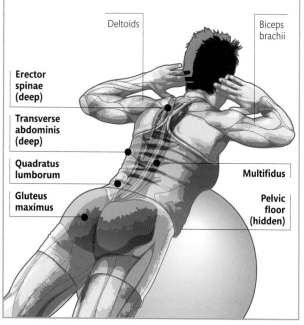

Deltoids

Biceps brachii

Erector spinae (deep)

Transverse abdominis (deep)

Quadratus lumborum

Multifidus

Gluteus maximus

Pelvic floor (hidden)

WARNING!

Before the exercise, check that the ball is the right size for your limb length. You should be able to touch the floor with straight arms when face down on the ball. Keep your movement controlled; if you straighten your torso too fast you risk compressing the vertebrae in your back and damaging your sciatic nerve. Do not pull your torso above the natural line of your spine – hyper-extending your back can be dangerous.

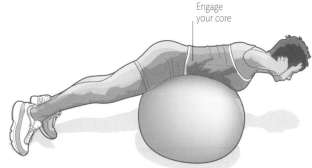

Engage your core

1 Lie on an exercise ball with your abs and upper thighs "wrapped" across it and your toes touching the floor.

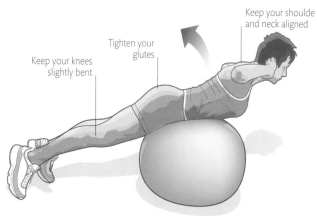

Keep your shoulder and neck aligned

Tighten your glutes

Keep your knees slightly bent

2 With the tips of your fingers touching the sides of your head, slowly straighten your body while breathing out, contracting your abs and glutes to control the movement.

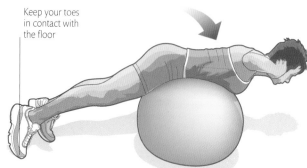

Keep your toes in contact with the floor

3 Gently and smoothly lower your upper body to the start position while breathing out.

MEDICINE BALL BRIDGE

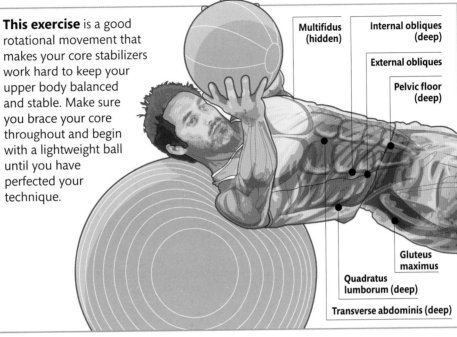

TARGET MUSCLES

- Transverse abdominis
- External obliques
- Internal obliques
- Pelvic floor
- Multifidus
- Quadratus lumborum
- Gluteus maximus

TARGET MOVEMENT

Rotation

DIFFICULTY LEVEL

This exercise is a good rotational movement that makes your core stabilizers work hard to keep your upper body balanced and stable. Make sure you brace your core throughout and begin with a lightweight ball until you have perfected your technique.

Multifidus (hidden)

Internal obliques (deep)

External obliques

Pelvic floor (deep)

Gluteus maximus

Quadratus lumborum (deep)

Transverse abdominis (deep)

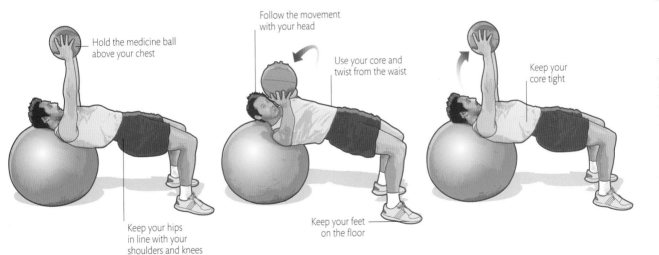

Hold the medicine ball above your chest

Keep your hips in line with your shoulders and knees

Follow the movement with your head

Use your core and twist from the waist

Keep your feet on the floor

Keep your core tight

1 Holding a medicine ball, carefully lie back against an exercise ball, with your upper body supported, your knees bent at right angles, and your feet firmly planted on the floor. Hold the ball above you with your arms straight.

2 Keeping your feet planted, your hips aligned, and your arms straight, rotate your torso to the right as far as possible, controlling the movement with your core and pivoting from your hips.

3 Pause at the edge of the movement, then rotate your torso back to the start position, keeping your core engaged. Repeat the movement to your left, then alternate sides for the required number of repetitions.

WALL SIDE THROW

TARGET MUSCLES	TARGET MOVEMENT
■ Transverse abdominis	
■ External obliques	
■ Internal obliques	
■ Pelvic floor	
■ Quadratus lumborum	Rotation

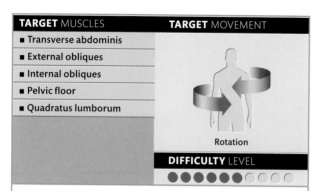

DIFFICULTY LEVEL

This powerful, dynamic exercise helps to build good rotational stability and control in your core, while also giving your upper body a good workout.

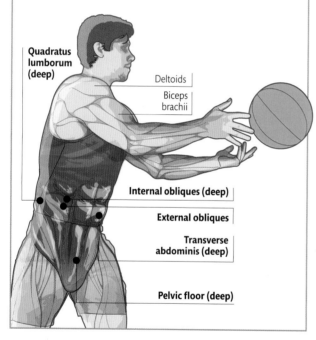

Quadratus lumborum (deep)

Deltoids

Biceps brachii

Internal obliques (deep)

External obliques

Transverse abdominis (deep)

Pelvic floor (deep)

1 Stand perpendicular to a wall around 1–1.5m (3–5ft) away, with your left foot closest to it. Grip the medicine ball at waist level and turn your torso to the right, keeping your hips, knees, and feet aligned.

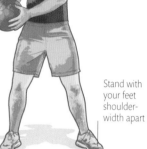

Stand with your feet shoulder-width apart

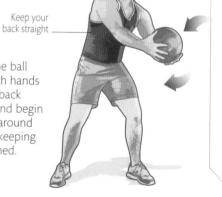

Keep your back straight

4 Catch the ball with both hands as it bounces back towards you and begin rotating back around to your right, keeping your hips aligned.

PROGRESSION 1

Removing the support of your feet focuses the movement on your hips, and makes the muscles work harder to stabilize your spine. Assume an upright kneeling position, and carry out the movement as in the main sequence, matching the number of repetitions for each side of your body.

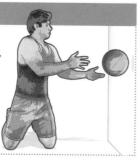

PROGRESSION 2

This further progression introduces more of a lateral movement to the arc of the ball, increasing the rotational stress on your body to make your core work even harder.

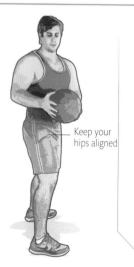

Keep your hips aligned

1 Stand facing a wall, around 1–1.5m (3–5ft) away. Hold the medicine ball at waist level and turn your torso to your right, pivoting from your hips.

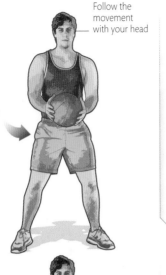

Follow the movement with your head

2 In one quick but controlled motion, rotate your torso to your left, controlling the movement with your hips, and holding the ball in front of you with your elbows aligned.

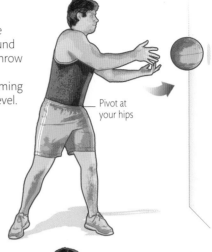

3 Continue the rotation around to your left, then throw the ball underarm against the wall, aiming for around chest level.

Pivot at your hips

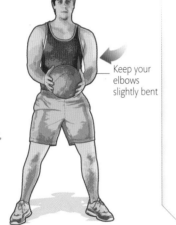

Keep your elbows slightly bent

5 Move the ball back around to the right in an arc, pivoting your torso from your hips.

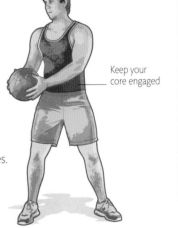

Keep your core engaged

6 Return to the start position. Pause briefly, then repeat as required before switching sides.

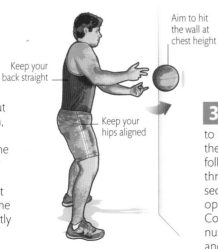

Keep your back straight

Aim to hit the wall at chest height

Keep your hips aligned

2 In one quick but smooth motion, rotate your torso to the left, controlling the movement with your hips, and throw the ball underarm against the wall, aiming for the area of the wall directly in front of you.

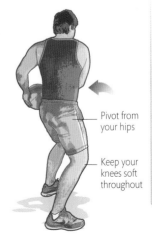

3 Continue rotating your torso around to the left, and catch the ball as you turn, following the movement through. Repeat the sequence in the opposite direction. Complete the desired number of repetitions and relax.

Pivot from your hips

Keep your knees soft throughout

SUSPENDED SINGLE-ARM CORE ROTATION

TARGET MUSCLES	**TARGET** MOVEMENT

TARGET MUSCLES
- Transverse abdominis
- External obliques
- Internal obliques
- Pelvic floor
- Erector spinae
- Multifidus
- Quadratus lumborum

TARGET MOVEMENT

Rotation

DIFFICULTY LEVEL

This rotational movement works the muscles of your obliques, abdominals, and back, while offering additional benefits to your shoulders and arms. It is important to keep your body aligned throughout and to repeat the same number of reps on both sides of your body.

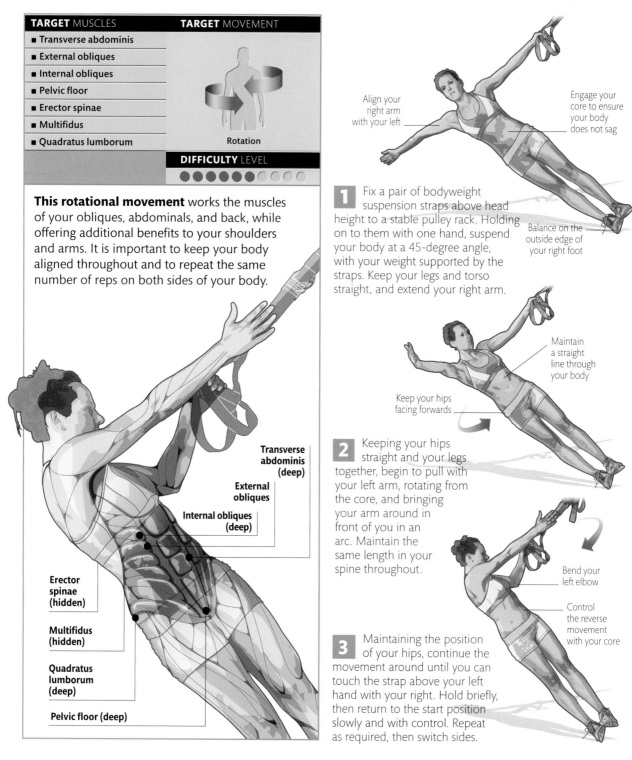

Transverse abdominis (deep)

External obliques

Internal obliques (deep)

Erector spinae (hidden)

Multifidus (hidden)

Quadratus lumborum (deep)

Pelvic floor (deep)

Align your right arm with your left

Engage your core to ensure your body does not sag

Balance on the outside edge of your right foot

1 Fix a pair of bodyweight suspension straps above head height to a stable pulley rack. Holding on to them with one hand, suspend your body at a 45-degree angle, with your weight supported by the straps. Keep your legs and torso straight, and extend your right arm.

Maintain a straight line through your body

Keep your hips facing forwards

2 Keeping your hips straight and your legs together, begin to pull with your left arm, rotating from the core, and bringing your arm around in front of you in an arc. Maintain the same length in your spine throughout.

Bend your left elbow

Control the reverse movement with your core

3 Maintaining the position of your hips, continue the movement around until you can touch the strap above your left hand with your right. Hold briefly, then return to the start position slowly and with control. Repeat as required, then switch sides.

SUSPENDED PENDULUM

TARGET MUSCLES	**TARGET** MOVEMENT
■ Transverse abdominis	
■ External obliques	
■ Internal obliques	
■ Pelvic floor	
■ Quadratus lumborum	
■ Gluteus maximus	

Complex

DIFFICULTY LEVEL

This challenging core exercise employs the resistance and instability of bodyweight suspension straps to rotate your core from a plank position (»pp.102–03). Good form is key, as is ensuring that you balance your movements on both sides.

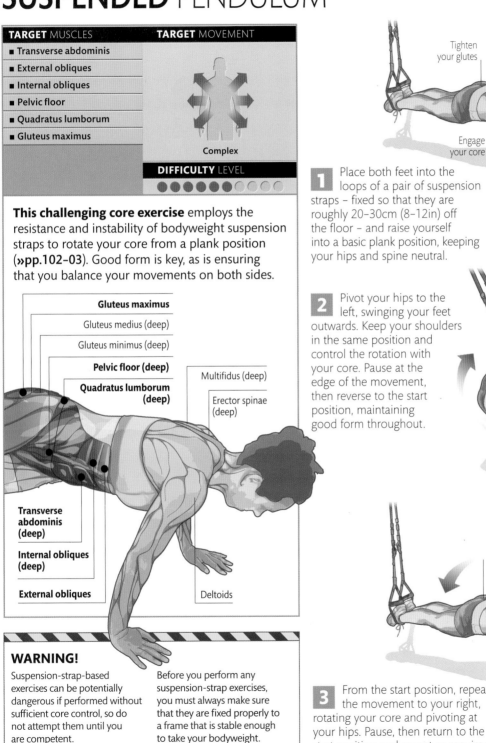

Gluteus maximus

Gluteus medius (deep)

Gluteus minimus (deep)

Pelvic floor (deep)

Quadratus lumborum (deep)

Multifidus (deep)

Erector spinae (deep)

Transverse abdominis (deep)

Internal obliques (deep)

External obliques

Deltoids

WARNING!

Suspension-strap-based exercises can be potentially dangerous if performed without sufficient core control, so do not attempt them until you are competent.

Before you perform any suspension-strap exercises, you must always make sure that they are fixed properly to a frame that is stable enough to take your bodyweight.

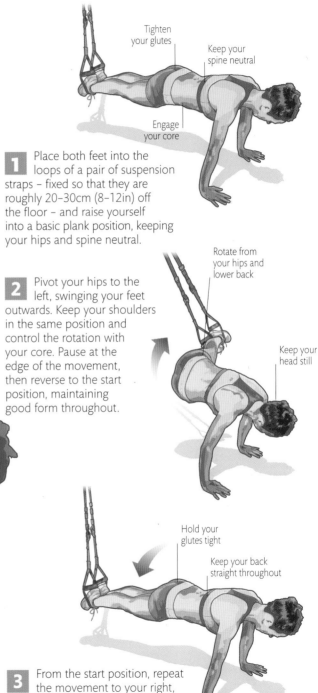

Tighten your glutes

Keep your spine neutral

Engage your core

1 Place both feet into the loops of a pair of suspension straps – fixed so that they are roughly 20–30cm (8–12in) off the floor – and raise yourself into a basic plank position, keeping your hips and spine neutral.

Rotate from your hips and lower back

Keep your head still

2 Pivot your hips to the left, swinging your feet outwards. Keep your shoulders in the same position and control the rotation with your core. Pause at the edge of the movement, then reverse to the start position, maintaining good form throughout.

Hold your glutes tight

Keep your back straight throughout

3 From the start position, repeat the movement to your right, rotating your core and pivoting at your hips. Pause, then return to the start position and repeat as required.

LONG-ARM BRIDGE PULL-OVER

TARGET MUSCLES	TARGET MOVEMENT
■ Transverse abdominis	
■ Pelvic floor	
■ Multifidus	
■ Quadratus lumborum	
■ Gluteus maximus	

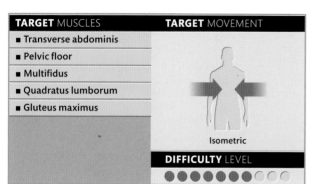

Isometric

DIFFICULTY LEVEL

This is an effective, though underused, core exercise. Good form is crucial to avoid straining the muscles of your shoulders and neck, so ensure you start with a weight you are comfortable with and focus on controlling the movement with your core.

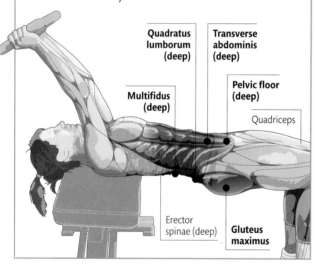

Quadratus lumborum (deep)

Transverse abdominis (deep)

Multifidus (deep)

Pelvic floor (deep)

Quadriceps

Erector spinae (deep)

Gluteus maximus

PROGRESSION

For a more challenging version of this movement, replace the bench with an exercise ball. This forces your core to work harder to compensate for the lack of stability. Holding the weight disc in front of you, carefully lie back against the exercise ball, keeping your knees bent and your feet flat. Perform the same movement as in the main sequence with good control.

1 Lie back against a weights bench so that it supports your shoulders. Position your feet flat on the floor and hip-width apart, and bend your knees at 90 degrees. Keep your hips up and aligned with the spine. Grip a weight disc and raise your arms above your chest.

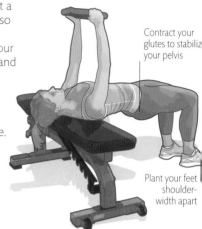

Contract your glutes to stabilize your pelvis

Plant your feet shoulder-width apart

Keep your arms aligned

Brace your core to maintain spine alignment

2 Holding your core tight and keeping your arms straight and elbows aligned, lift the weight disc over your head with a slow and controlled movement.

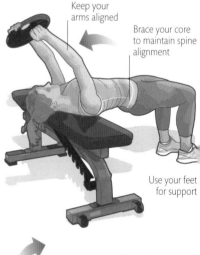

Use your feet for support

Control the movement with your core

3 Continue the movement so that your arms are almost in line with your body, but avoid straining. Pause briefly, then reverse the movement to the start position with a slow, controlled motion.

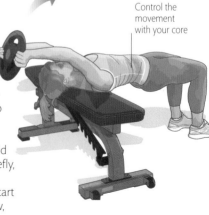

KETTLEBELL SWING

TARGET MUSCLES	TARGET MOVEMENT
■ Rectus abdominis	
■ Transverse abdominis	
■ Pelvic floor	
■ Hip flexors	
■ Erector spinae	
■ Multifidus	
■ Quadratus lumborum	Isometric
■ Gluteus minimus/medius	**DIFFICULTY** LEVEL
■ Gluteus maximus	

This whole-body exercise works the muscles of your glutes, lower back, and hips. Allow the kettlebell to hang loosely from your arms and generate the force of the movement from your hips, rather than trying to "muscle" the weight up with your upper body.

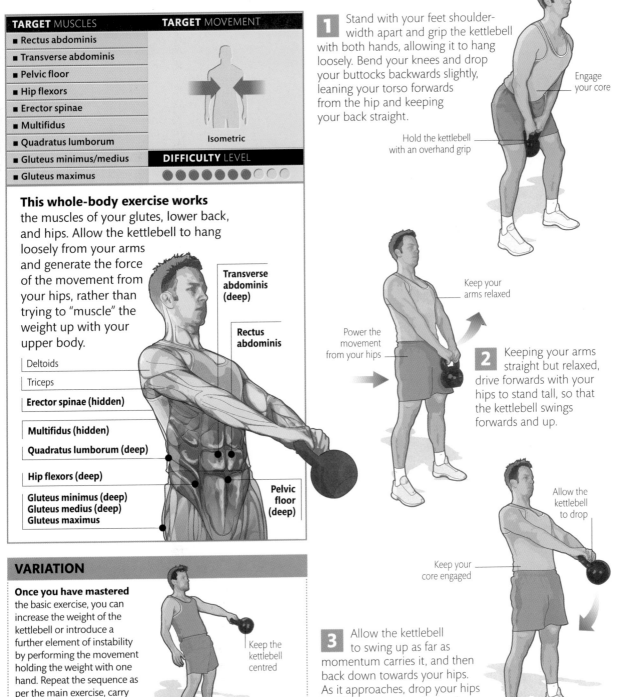

Deltoids

Triceps

Erector spinae (hidden)

Multifidus (hidden)

Quadratus lumborum (deep)

Hip flexors (deep)

Gluteus minimus (deep)
Gluteus medius (deep)
Gluteus maximus

Transverse abdominis (deep)

Rectus abdominis

Pelvic floor (deep)

1 Stand with your feet shoulder-width apart and grip the kettlebell with both hands, allowing it to hang loosely. Bend your knees and drop your buttocks backwards slightly, leaning your torso forwards from the hip and keeping your back straight.

Engage your core

Hold the kettlebell with an overhand grip

Keep your arms relaxed

Power the movement from your hips

2 Keeping your arms straight but relaxed, drive forwards with your hips to stand tall, so that the kettlebell swings forwards and up.

Allow the kettlebell to drop

Keep your core engaged

3 Allow the kettlebell to swing up as far as momentum carries it, and then back down towards your hips. As it approaches, drop your hips and lean your torso forwards, and keeping your back straight, to return to the start position.

VARIATION

Once you have mastered the basic exercise, you can increase the weight of the kettlebell or introduce a further element of instability by performing the movement holding the weight with one hand. Repeat the sequence as per the main exercise, carry out the desired number of reps, then switch hands.

Keep the kettlebell centred

EXERCISE BALL KNEE TUCK

TARGET MUSCLES	TARGET MOVEMENT
▪ Rectus abdominis	
▪ Transverse abdominis	
▪ Pelvic floor	
▪ Erector spinae	
▪ Multifidus	
▪ Quadratus lumborum	
▪ Gluteus medius	Isometric
▪ Gluteus maximus	
	DIFFICULTY LEVEL

This relatively advanced exercise demands great balance and control. It works the core muscles that flex your hips and also stresses your abdominals, spinal stabilizers, and glutes.

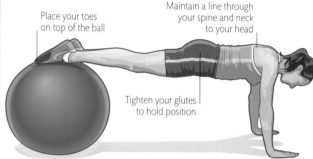

Place your toes on top of the ball

Maintain a line through your spine and neck to your head

Tighten your glutes to hold position

1 Position the tops of your feet on an exercise ball and assume a press-up position, keeping your hands flat on the floor and your feet elevated on the ball. Align your head with your spine.

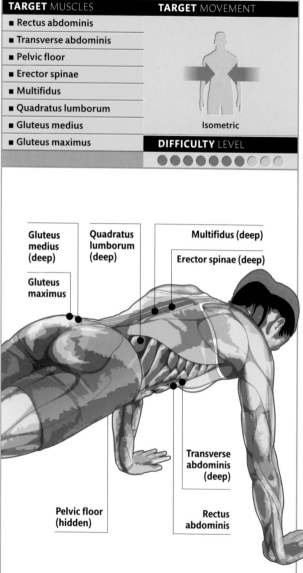

Gluteus medius (deep)

Quadratus lumborum (deep)

Multifidus (deep)

Erector spinae (deep)

Gluteus maximus

Transverse abdominis (deep)

Pelvic floor (hidden)

Rectus abdominis

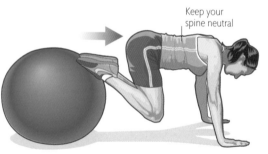

Keep your spine neutral

2 Draw your knees towards your chest, keeping your shoulders stable and your back straight as the ball rolls forwards.

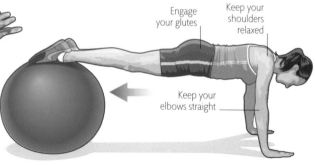

Engage your glutes

Keep your shoulders relaxed

Keep your elbows straight

3 Reverse the movement to return to the start position, controlling the motion with your core and keeping your back and neck in a neutral position.

WARNING!

Performing this exercise with good technique is important to avoid injury. Never allow your hips or lower back to sag, as this will place stress on your back – keeping your glutes tight will help to keep your back straight. Choose a ball that has a diameter about the same as the length of your arm. This should help to ensure your back is parallel to the floor when you assume the press-up position.

CORE BOARD ROTATION

TARGET MUSCLES	TARGET MOVEMENT
■ Transverse abdominis	
■ Internal obliques	
■ Pelvic floor	
■ Erector spinae	
■ Multifidus	
■ Gluteus medius	
■ Gluteus maximus	Isometric

DIFFICULTY LEVEL

This challenging exercise is essentially a variation on the plank, with the added difficulties of instability and small rotational movements to make your core work even harder. To begin with, you may find it easier to get into position with your knees on the ground.

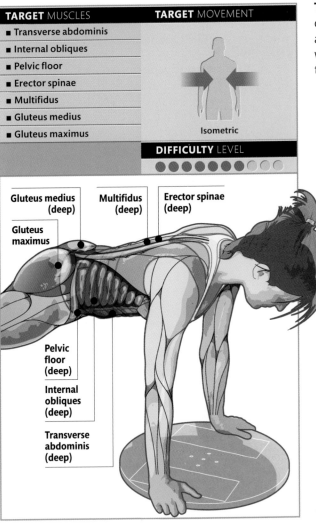

Gluteus medius (deep)

Multifidus (deep)

Erector spinae (deep)

Gluteus maximus

Pelvic floor (deep)

Internal obliques (deep)

Transverse abdominis (deep)

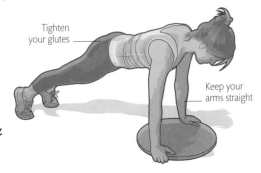

Tighten your glutes

Keep your arms straight

1 Carefully gripping either side of a core board, engage your core and assume a normal plank position.

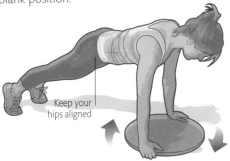

Keep your hips aligned

2 Rotate the core board 90 degrees to the right, keeping your shoulders aligned, and holding your body in the plank position with your core braced and your glutes tight.

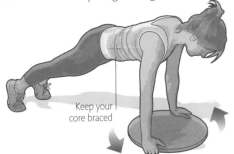

Keep your core braced

3 Pause, then rotate the board back to the start position with a slow, controlled movement. Repeat the sequence in the opposite direction.

PROGRESSION

Once you have mastered the basic exercise, try tilting the board rather than rotating it to increase the level of instability and make your core work harder. Lift with one hand and place the other flat on the upper surface of the board, rather than gripping it, to avoid crushing your fingers.

Maintain a straight back

Keep your right arm straight and your right hand flat

EXERCISE BALL ROLL-OUT

TARGET MUSCLES	TARGET MOVEMENT
■ Transverse abdominis	
■ Pelvic floor	
■ Erector spinae	
■ Multifidus	
■ Gluteus maximus	Complex

DIFFICULTY LEVEL

In a similar way to the plank, this excellent core exercise builds stability and strength in the muscles of your abdomen and lower back, with the added challenge of forward movement, working your upper back and shoulder stability.

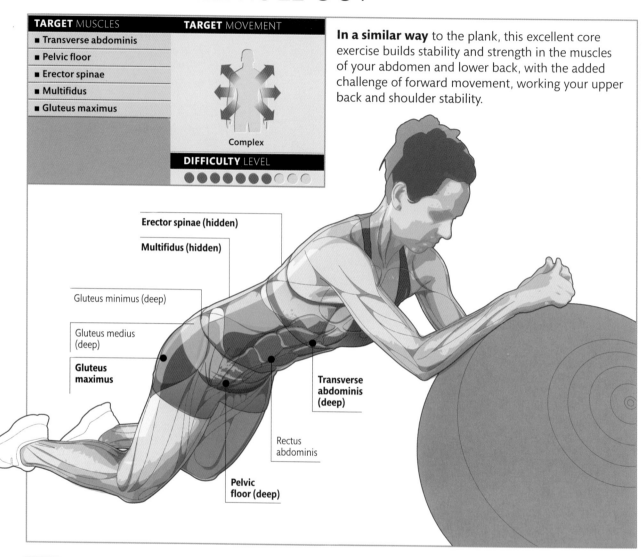

Erector spinae (hidden)

Multifidus (hidden)

Gluteus minimus (deep)

Gluteus medius (deep)

Gluteus maximus

Transverse abdominis (deep)

Rectus abdominis

Pelvic floor (deep)

WARNING!

While this is a great exercise for building your core, it requires a good level of existing core strength and stability to perform. It is important to keep your back straight throughout, with your shoulders and hips aligned. To begin with, only roll the ball out as far as you can comfortably maintain good form, and never allow your lower back to sag,

as this can potentially cause back strain or similar injuries. Engaging your gluteal muscles will help you hold your pelvis in position, and you can also place a towel beneath your knees if you find they become painful during the roll-out. You should practise and perfect the basic movement before you try the variation or progression.

PROGRESSION

To increase the instability and the intensity of this exercise, you can perform it with your knees balanced on a stability disc rather than on the floor. Carefully roll the exercise ball forwards and backwards as before, but use your core to keep your balance on the stability disc.

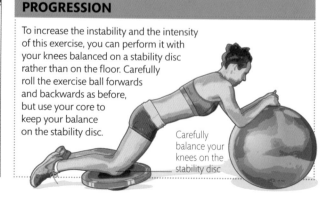

Carefully balance your knees on the stability disc

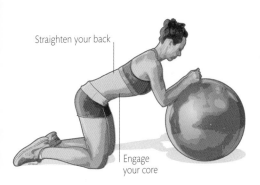

Straighten your back

Engage your core

1 Kneel down with an exercise ball positioned in front of you. Engaging your core and straightening your back, rest your hands and lower arms on the top of the ball.

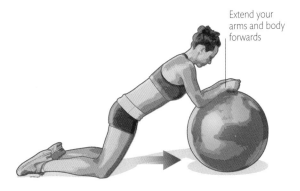

Extend your arms and body forwards

2 Roll the ball forwards by extending your arms, and follow it with your upper body as far as you can, keeping your core tight, your back straight, and shoulders stable.

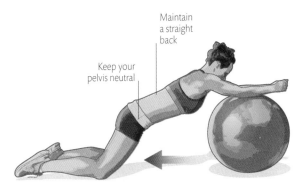

Maintain a straight back

Keep your pelvis neutral

3 Extend the movement, hold for a few seconds, and then reverse to the start position, controlling the movement of the ball with your core.

VARIATION

Using a barbell instead of an exercise ball places slightly different demands on your core, due to the lowered body position and the increased range of movement it allows.

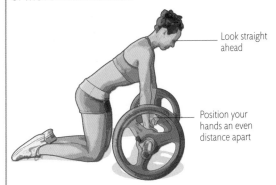

Look straight ahead

Position your hands an even distance apart

1 Kneel with a barbell in front of you. Using an overhand grip, place both of your hands on the bar, shoulder-width apart.

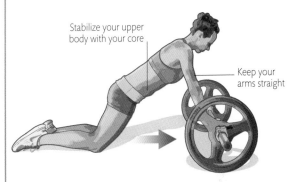

Stabilize your upper body with your core

Keep your arms straight

2 Engaging your core and keeping your back straight, begin to roll the bar forwards, keeping your shoulders stable.

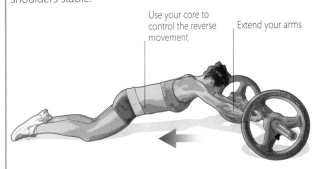

Use your core to control the reverse movement

Extend your arms

3 Extend the movement until your back is almost parallel to the floor, pause, then reverse the movement slowly and under control to return to the start position.

SUSPENDED CRUNCH

TARGET MUSCLES	TARGET MOVEMENT
■ Rectus abdominis	
■ Transverse abdominis	
■ Internal obliques	
■ Pelvic floor	
■ Hip flexors	
■ Erector spinae	
■ Multifidus	
■ Quadratus lumborum	

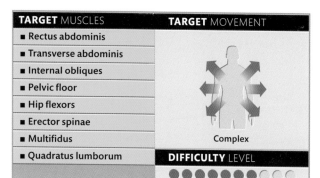

Complex

DIFFICULTY LEVEL

●●●●●●●●○○○

This highly taxing form of the crunch (»p.72) uses suspension straps, challenging your core to maintain stability during the movement.

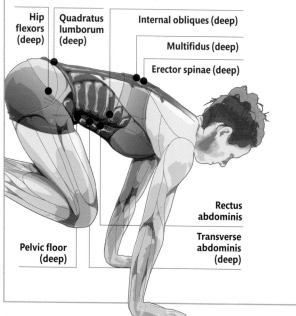

Hip flexors (deep)

Quadratus lumborum (deep)

Internal obliques (deep)

Multifidus (deep)

Erector spinae (deep)

Rectus abdominis

Transverse abdominis (deep)

Pelvic floor (deep)

PROGRESSION

Performing the exercise in a pike position makes it even harder for your core muscles to stabilize your torso and legs. As with the main exercise, do not attempt this unless you have excellent core strength. Lift your hips and move your feet and legs (in a straight line) towards your upper body, essentially forming a narrow pike.

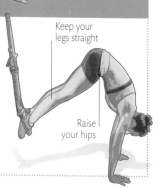

Keep your legs straight

Raise your hips

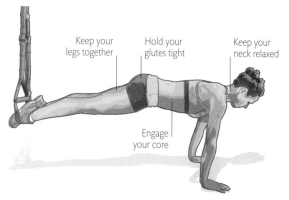

Keep your legs together

Hold your glutes tight

Keep your neck relaxed

Engage your core

1 Fix a pair of bodyweight suspension straps to a stable rack so they are approximately 20–30cm (8–12in) above the floor. Insert your feet into the loops and adopt the plank position (»pp.102–03), with your core engaged.

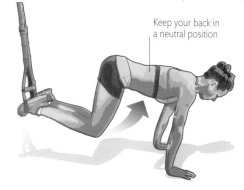

Keep your back in a neutral position

2 Keeping your feet firmly in the loops, and your core engaged, lift your hips and pull your knees smoothly towards your chest in a reverse crunch movement.

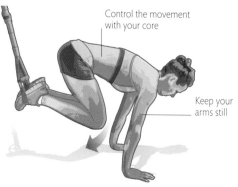

Control the movement with your core

Keep your arms still

3 Bring your knees as close as you can towards your chest to complete the movement. Hold briefly, then reverse the sequence to return to the starting position.

SUSPENDED OBLIQUE CRUNCH

TARGET MUSCLES	TARGET MOVEMENT
■ Transverse abdominis	
■ External obliques	
■ Internal obliques	
■ Pelvic floor	
■ Hip flexors	
■ Erector spinae	
■ Multifidus	
■ Quadratus lumborum	Complex

DIFFICULTY LEVEL

Similar to the suspended pendulum (**»p.127**), this exercise works your core using the instability produced by suspension straps. As before, make sure you maintain good form throughout, and match the movements on either side of your body.

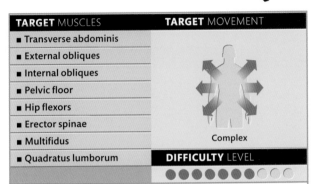

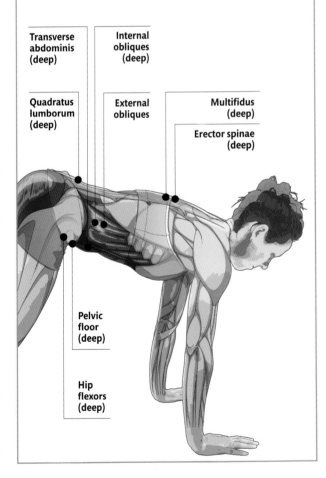

Transverse abdominis (deep)

Internal obliques (deep)

Quadratus lumborum (deep)

External obliques

Multifidus (deep)

Erector spinae (deep)

Pelvic floor (deep)

Hip flexors (deep)

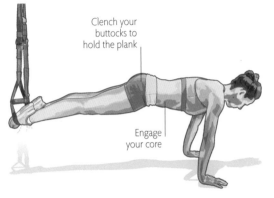

Clench your buttocks to hold the plank

Engage your core

1 Fix a pair of bodyweight suspension straps in the same way as for the suspended crunch (opposite), secure your feet and raise your body into a plank (**»pp.102–03**).

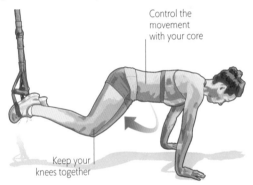

Control the movement with your core

Keep your knees together

2 Pivot your hips to the right, controlling the rotation with the core. As you do so, bend your knees, bringing them up to the right of your chest.

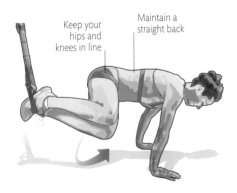

Keep your hips and knees in line

Maintain a straight back

3 Continue bending your knees up towards the right of your chest with a crunching motion. Hold briefly at the edge of the movement, then slowly return to the start position. Repeat as required, then switch sides.

MEDICINE BALL CHOP

TARGET MUSCLES	TARGET MOVEMENT

TARGET MUSCLES
- Transverse abdominis
- External obliques
- Internal obliques
- Pelvic floor
- Erector spinae
- Multifidus
- Quadratus lumborum
- Gluteus maximus

TARGET MOVEMENT

Complex

DIFFICULTY LEVEL

This exercise is good for developing rotational strength and spinal control, while offering additional benefits to the muscles of your legs and shoulders. Always repeat the same number of reps on both sides.

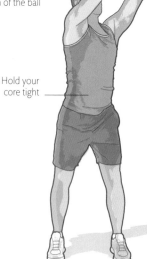

Gaze in the direction of the ball

Hold your core tight

1 Holding a medicine ball in both hands, stand with your legs shoulder-width apart. Engaging your core, grip the ball and raise your arms up and to your left, holding it above your left shoulder.

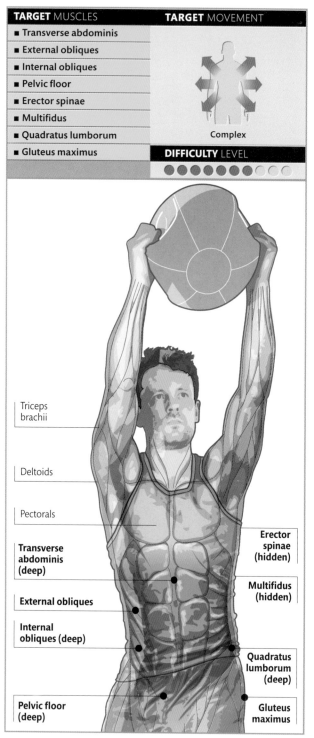

Triceps brachii

Deltoids

Pectorals

Transverse abdominis (deep)

External obliques

Internal obliques (deep)

Pelvic floor (deep)

Erector spinae (hidden)

Multifidus (hidden)

Quadratus lumborum (deep)

Gluteus maximus

Look straight ahead

Bend at your hips

2 Keeping your arms straight, slowly bring the ball down and in front of you across your torso, bending your knees and dropping back with your hips into a half-squat as you do so.

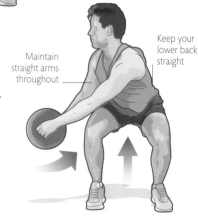

Keep your lower back straight

Maintain straight arms throughout

3 Maintaining the half-squat position, bring the ball down and to your right, following the direction of the movement with your gaze. Pause, then slowly reverse the exercise to return to the start position. Repeat as required, then switch sides.

LAWNMOWER

TARGET MUSCLES	TARGET MOVEMENT
■ External obliques	
■ Internal obliques	
■ Pelvic floor	
■ Erector spinae	
■ Multifidus	
■ Quadratus lumborum	
■ Gluteus minimus	Complex
■ Gluteus medius	**DIFFICULTY** LEVEL
■ Gluteus maximus	

An excellent core rotation exercise, the lawnmower uses a similar movement to the medicine ball chop (opposite) but with a greater range and the additional challenge of holding the weight in one hand. It can take a while to perfect your form, so practise in front of a mirror until you can execute it with confidence.

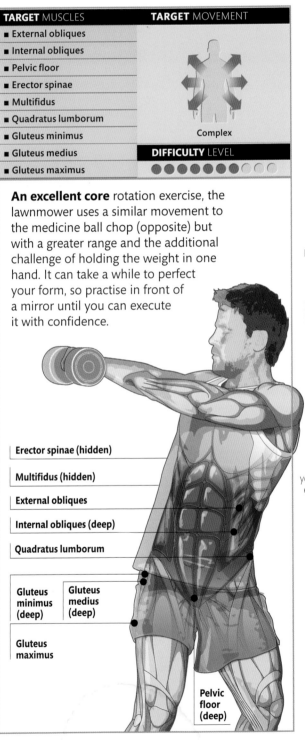

Erector spinae (hidden)

Multifidus (hidden)

External obliques

Internal obliques (deep)

Quadratus lumborum

Gluteus minimus (deep)   Gluteus medius (deep)

Gluteus maximus

Pelvic floor (deep)

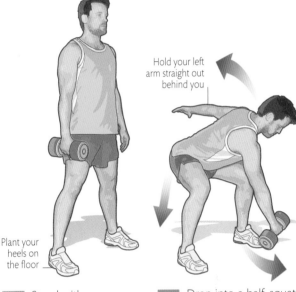

Plant your heels on the floor

Hold your left arm straight out behind you

1 Stand with your feet slightly more than shoulder-width apart, with a dumbbell in your right hand.

2 Drop into a half-squat and, leaning forwards from your waist, lower the dumbbell across your legs in front of your left ankle.

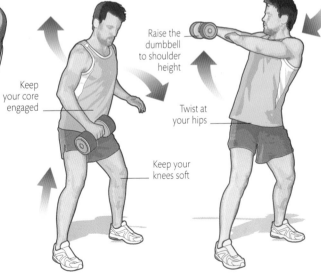

Keep your core engaged

Raise the dumbbell to shoulder height

Twist at your hips

Keep your knees soft

3 Pulling the dumbbell up and across your torso, straighten your legs, rotate the upper body, and swing your left arm forwards.

4 Pull the weight up to shoulder level, bringing your left arm across your body as you do so. Pause, then return to the start. Switch arms.

ADVANCED

The exercises in this section involve challenging and complex movements that require excellent all-round core strength, stability, and mobility to perform correctly. It is therefore important that you do not attempt any of them until you have mastered the exercises in the previous sections and can perform them confidently with optimum form and technique.

GHD SIT-UP

TARGET MUSCLES	TARGET MOVEMENT
■ Rectus abdominis	
■ Transverse abdominis	
■ Pelvic floor	
■ Hip flexors	
■ Erector spinae	
■ Multifidus	Flexion

DIFFICULTY LEVEL

This advanced version of a basic sit-up offers a greater challenge to your abs and lower back, and requires good flexibility in your hips.

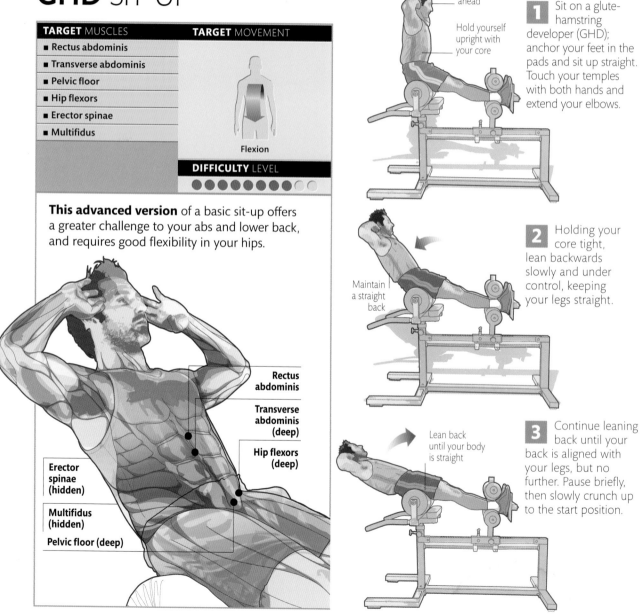

Rectus abdominis

Transverse abdominis (deep)

Hip flexors (deep)

Erector spinae (hidden)

Multifidus (hidden)

Pelvic floor (deep)

Look straight ahead

Hold yourself upright with your core

1 Sit on a glute-hamstring developer (GHD); anchor your feet in the pads and sit up straight. Touch your temples with both hands and extend your elbows.

Maintain a straight back

2 Holding your core tight, lean backwards slowly and under control, keeping your legs straight.

Lean back until your body is straight

3 Continue leaning back until your back is aligned with your legs, but no further. Pause briefly, then slowly crunch up to the start position.

PIKE

<table>
<tr><td colspan="2">TARGET MUSCLES</td></tr>
</table>

TARGET MUSCLES
- Rectus abdominis
- Transverse abdominis
- Pelvic floor
- Hip flexors

TARGET MOVEMENT

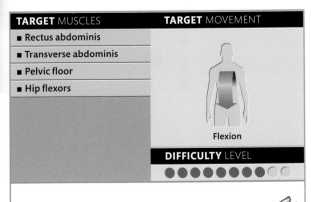

Flexion

DIFFICULTY LEVEL

This exercise demands excellent core control and flexibility, and takes practice to perfect. It is important to focus on good form and control the upwards and downwards phases with your core, rather than straining with your legs or back, which can cause injury.

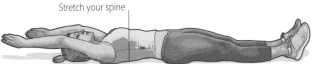

Stretch your spine

1 Lie flat on the floor with your legs together and your arms stretched above your head, shoulder-width apart, palms facing inwards.

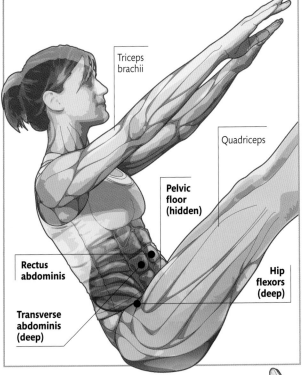

Triceps brachii

Quadriceps

Pelvic floor (hidden)

Rectus abdominis

Hip flexors (deep)

Transverse abdominis (deep)

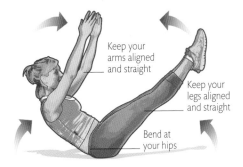

Keep your arms aligned and straight

Keep your legs aligned and straight

Bend at your hips

2 Using your core to drive the movement, raise your legs and upper body off the floor at the same time, keeping them straight, and bring your arms over in an arc towards your feet.

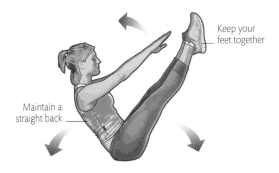

Keep your feet together

Maintain a straight back

3 Continue the movement to form a "V" shape, with your back and legs straight, and stretch your arms towards your toes. Hold briefly, then reverse the movement to the start position, controlling it with your core.

PROGRESSION

Once you have mastered the basic movement, you can try the exercise while holding a small weight, such as a kettlebell, to make the exercise harder. As you improve you can increase the amount of weight in increments.

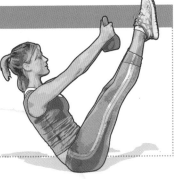

STICK CRUNCH

TARGET MUSCLES

- Rectus abdominis
- Transverse abdominis
- Pelvic floor
- Hip flexors
- Erector spinae
- Gluteus maximus

TARGET MOVEMENT

Flexion

DIFFICULTY LEVEL

This challenging exercise is a development of the V sit-up (**»p.93**), and requires excellent core stability to master. To begin with, practise using the variation below, taking the stick as far towards your toes as you can, focusing on perfecting your form, before attempting the full stick crunch in bare feet. A broomstick handle or similar is ideal for the exercise.

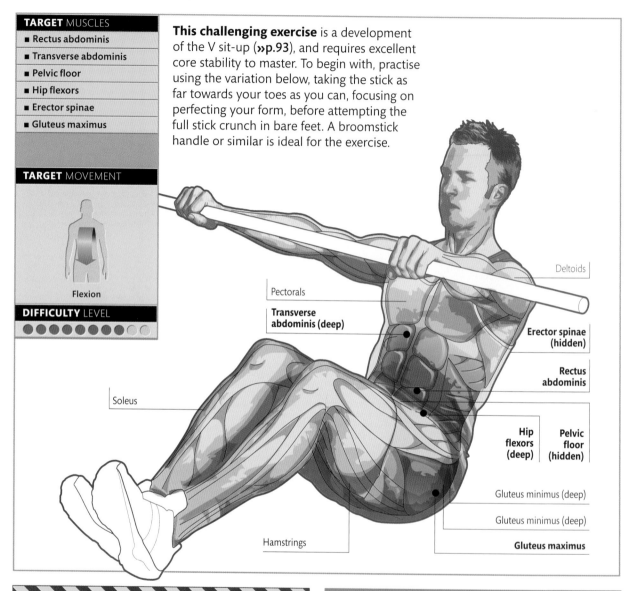

Deltoids

Pectorals

Transverse abdominis (deep)

Erector spinae (hidden)

Rectus abdominis

Soleus

Hip flexors (deep)

Pelvic floor (hidden)

Gluteus minimus (deep)

Gluteus minimus (deep)

Hamstrings

Gluteus maximus

WARNING!

This is an advanced exercise that requires a high level of core stability, strength, and mobility to perform correctly. So, you should not attempt it without first mastering exercises in the earlier sections of the book – particularly those involving similar movements such as the V leg-raise and V sit-up (**»pp.92–93**). Good form is key, because poor technique can result in back strain or related injuries, so focus on perfecting your technique to begin with, moving the stick only as far as it is comfortable to do so.

VARIATION

If you find the main exercise too hard, practise the first phase of the movement only — that is bringing the stick as far as you can down your shins towards your toes. Focus on developing good form and movement. You can attempt the full movement without shoes on. This reduces the clearance over your feet by 1–2cm (⅜–⅝in), making it slightly easier.

1 Grasping the stick with an overhand grip, your hands slightly wider than shoulder-width apart, lie on your back. Engaging your core, lift the stick.

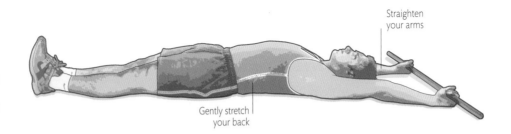

Straighten your arms

Gently stretch your back

2 Keeping your core tight, and your feet together, raise your knees towards your chest and crunch up with the upper body. Bring the stick over your head towards your knees as you do so.

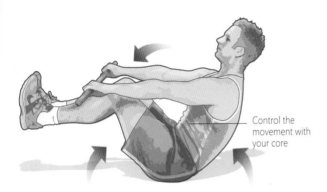

Control the movement with your core

3 Continue the crunch with a smooth, controlled movement, pulling your knees into your chest, and bring the stick down and around the soles of your feet without touching them.

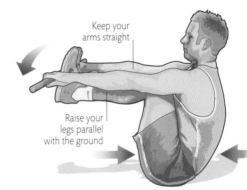

Keep your arms straight

Raise your legs parallel with the ground

4 Still bracing your core, bring the stick back under your legs, straightening your knees and leaning back with your torso, with a smooth, controlled movement, keeping your back straight.

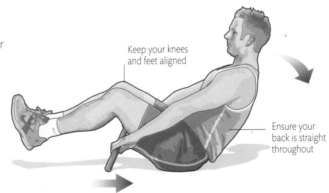

Keep your knees and feet aligned

Ensure your back is straight throughout

5 Continue the movement until your upper body is on the floor, and the stick is beneath your lower buttocks. Keep your legs straight and your feet slightly off the ground. Hold briefly, then reverse the sequence to the start position.

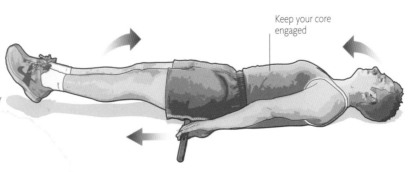

Keep your core engaged

EXERCISE BALL JACK-KNIFE

TARGET MUSCLES	TARGET MOVEMENT
■ Rectus abdominis	
■ Transverse abdominis	
■ Pelvic floor	
■ Erector spinae	
■ Quadratus lumborum	
■ Gluteus maximus	Flexion

DIFFICULTY LEVEL

This difficult core flexion exercise demands excellent core stability, balance, and control to perform correctly. Because the movement can potentially cause injury when performed with poor form, you should only attempt it once you have mastered a good range of basic core exercises.

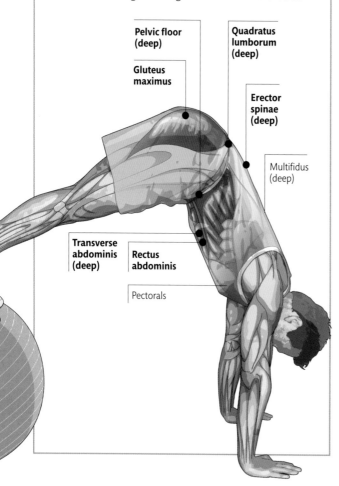

Pelvic floor (deep)

Quadratus lumborum (deep)

Gluteus maximus

Erector spinae (deep)

Multifidus (deep)

Transverse abdominis (deep)

Rectus abdominis

Pectorals

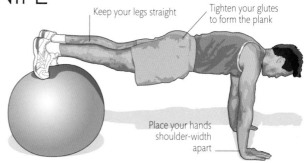

Keep your legs straight

Tighten your glutes to form the plank

Place your hands shoulder-width apart

1 Assume a plank (**»pp.102–03**), with your hands on the floor below your shoulders and your feet on an exercise ball. Keep your elbows straight, but not locked, your shoulders relaxed, and the head supported by neck muscles. Hold your back straight and ensure your pelvis is not tipping downwards.

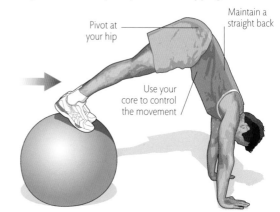

Pivot at your hip

Maintain a straight back

Use your core to control the movement

2 Keeping your body straight and your hands fixed in position, slowly lift from your lower abdominals, bending at the hip. Push as far as you can, keeping control of the movement with your core.

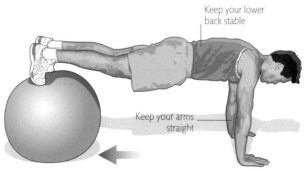

Keep your lower back stable

Keep your arms straight

3 Hold the position for a few seconds, then return to the start position with a slow, controlled movement.

GHD BACK EXTENSION

TARGET MUSCLES	TARGET MOVEMENT
■ Transverse abdominis	
■ Pelvic floor	
■ Erector spinae	
■ Multifidus	
■ Gluteus maximus	

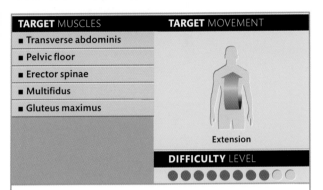

Extension

DIFFICULTY LEVEL

Essentially an advanced version of the basic dorsal raise (**»pp.76–77**),this exercise is harder than it looks. Using a glute–hamstring developer (GHD) machine, the movement targets the muscles of your spine, lower back, and glutes in the same way, but demands a much greater level of flexibility in your hips and hamstrings.

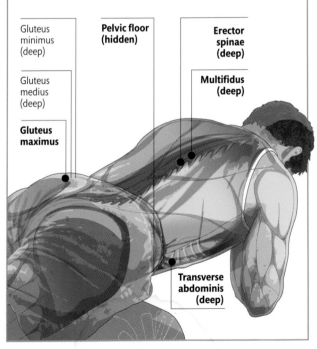

Gluteus minimus (deep)

Pelvic floor (hidden)

Erector spinae (deep)

Gluteus medius (deep)

Multifidus (deep)

Gluteus maximus

Transverse abdominis (deep)

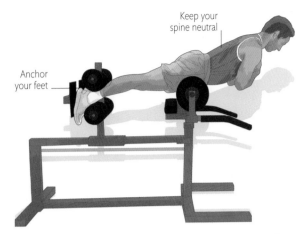

Keep your spine neutral

Anchor your feet

1 Position yourself on the GHD machine, with your feet anchored in the foot supports. With your spine in a neutral position, cross your hands over your chest.

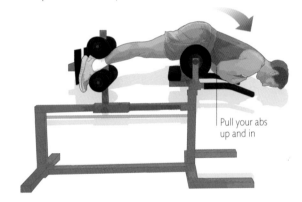

Pull your abs up and in

2 Flexing at your hips, drop your upper body slowly towards the floor, using your core to control the movement. Keep your arms tucked in and your legs straight.

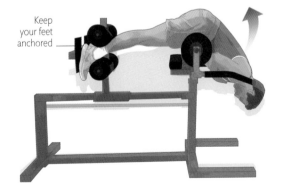

Keep your feet anchored

3 Bend downwards until the flexibility of your hamstrings restricts further movement. Maintaining good form, return to the start position, being careful not to extend beyond that point.

PULLEY CHOP

TARGET MUSCLES	TARGET MOVEMENT
■ Rectus abdominis	
■ Transverse abdominis	
■ External obliques	
■ Internal obliques	
■ Pelvic floor	
■ Quadratus lumborum	Rotation

DIFFICULTY LEVEL

The pulley chop is a powerful core-rotational exercise that is excellent for improving spinal control and stability, and building rotational strength. It can be partnered with the pulley lift (**»pp.146–47**).

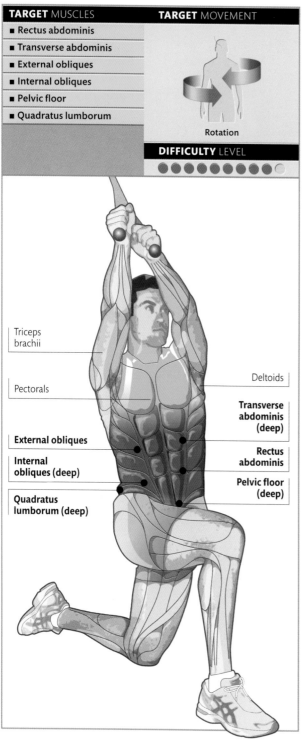

Triceps brachii

Pectorals

External obliques

Internal obliques (deep)

Quadratus lumborum (deep)

Deltoids

Transverse abdominis (deep)

Rectus abdominis

Pelvic floor (deep)

1 Assume a split kneeling position with a pulley cable machine to your right. Extend your right leg in front of you so that your knee is bent at 90 degrees and your foot is flat on the floor. Keeping your back straight, align your back, shoulders, hips, and knees. Grasp the handles of the cable with your arms straight.

Bend your leg at a right angle

2 Engaging your core, pull the cable down and across your body in a smooth, controlled movement, bending your elbows as you reach the mid-point of your chest.

Keep your shoulders straight

Engage your core

Keep your foot flat on the floor

3 Keeping the cable close to your body, push down with your arms to finish the movement. Hold briefly and return to the start position. Swap sides.

Keep your core engaged throughout

Keep your hips aligned with your knees

PROGRESSION 1

Performing the chop while standing makes your core muscles work harder to generate rotational power.

Keep your back straight, and avoid trying to "muscle" the movement down with your arm or shoulders.

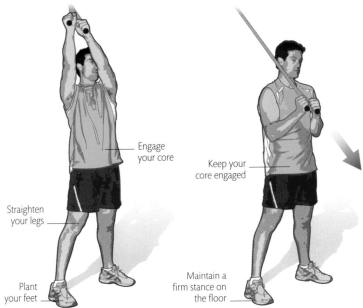

Engage your core

Straighten your legs

Plant your feet

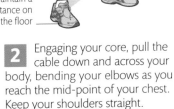

Keep your core engaged

Maintain a firm stance on the floor

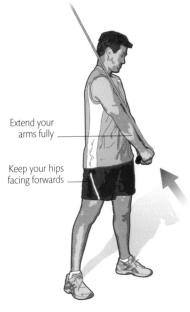

Extend your arms fully

Keep your hips facing forwards

1 Stand with the pulley to your right, keeping your back and legs straight, and your shoulders and hips aligned. Keeping your arms extended, grasp the cable handles.

2 Engaging your core, pull the cable down and across your body, bending your elbows as you reach the mid-point of your chest. Keep your shoulders straight.

3 Keeping the cable close to your body, push down with your arms to finish the movement. Hold briefly and return to the start position. Switch sides.

PROGRESSION 2

Performing the pulley chop movement in a scissors stance (a half-lunge position) adds an element of rotational instability, which increases the stresses on your core muscles, challenging them to work harder to keep you balanced. With the pulley machine to your right, take hold of the cable handles and assume a scissors stance. Follow the sequence as above, keeping your back straight and your core engaged, for the desired number of repetitions. Relax then switch sides, making sure you perform the same number of repetitions.

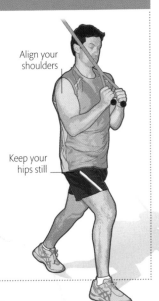

Align your shoulders

Keep your hips still

PROGRESSION 3

Adopting a full-lunge position to perform the pulley chop creates an even greater level of instability, and places additional rotational stress on the deep muscles of your spine and abdomen. Standing with the pulley machine to your right, grasp the pulley handles and drop into the lunge position, keeping your back straight and your core engaged. Follow the sequence as above for the desired number of repetitions, then swap sides, being sure to carry out the same number of movements.

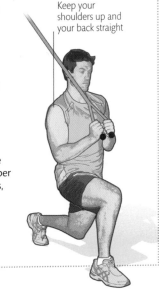

Keep your shoulders up and your back straight

PULLEY LIFT

TARGET MUSCLES	**TARGET** MOVEMENT
■ Transverse abdominis	
■ External obliques	
■ Internal obliques	
■ Pelvic floor	
■ Multifidus	
■ Quadratus lumborum	Rotation

DIFFICULTY LEVEL

The pulley lift is an excellent partner exercise to the pulley chop (**»pp.144–45**). A powerful and versatile movement, it improves rotational strength and spinal control and stability.

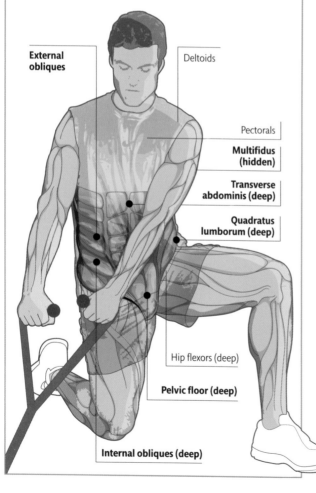

External obliques

Deltoids

Pectorals

Multifidus (hidden)

Transverse abdominis (deep)

Quadratus lumborum (deep)

Hip flexors (deep)

Pelvic floor (deep)

Internal obliques (deep)

1 Kneel down with a pulley to your right. Position yourself with your left knee bent at 90 degrees and your right knee on the floor. Keep your back straight with both shoulders and hips in line. Take hold of the pulley handle with both hands, keeping your arms straight.

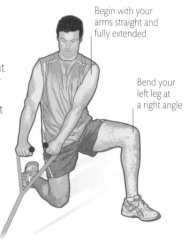

Begin with your arms straight and fully extended

Bend your left leg at a right angle

2 Pull the cable up and into your chest with both hands, bending at your elbows and keeping the cable taut and close to your body, controlling the movement with your core.

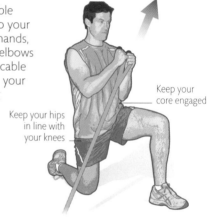

Keep your hips in line with your knees

Keep your core engaged

3 Following the direction of the pull across your upper body, push up with your hands until your arms are straight and fully extended. Hold briefly at the top of the movement, then return to the start position, and switch sides.

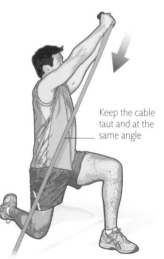

Keep the cable taut and at the same angle

PROGRESSION 1

Performing the lift in a standing position makes the muscles of your core work harder to generate rotational power. Be careful to carry out the movement in a smooth, controlled action.

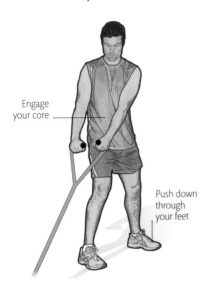

Engage your core

Push down through your feet

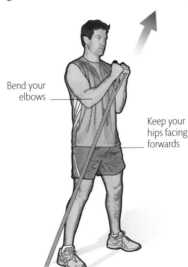

Bend your elbows

Keep your hips facing forwards

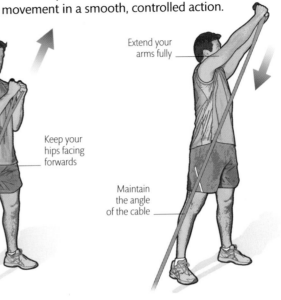

Extend your arms fully

Maintain the angle of the cable

1 Stand with the pulley to your right and your feet shoulder-width apart. With your back straight and your shoulders, hips, knees, and ankles aligned, grasp the pulley handle with both hands, on straight arms.

2 Pull the cable up and into your chest with both of your hands bending at the elbows. Remember to control the movement with your core, keeping the cable taut and close to your body.

3 Following the direction of the pull across your upper body, push up with your hands until your arms are straight and fully extended. Hold briefly at the top, then return to the start position and switch sides.

PROGRESSION 2

Carrying out the pulley lift in a scissors stance (a half-lunge position) adds an element of rotational instability, placing extra rotational stress on the deep muscles of your spine and abdomen. Assume a scissors stance with the pulley machine to your right and take hold of the cable handles. Keeping your back straight and your core engaged, follow the sequence as above for the desired number of repetitions, then swap sides, being sure to carry out the same number of movements.

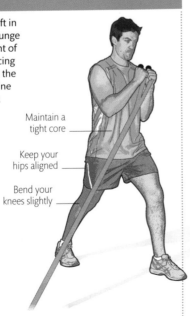

Maintain a tight core

Keep your hips aligned

Bend your knees slightly

PROGRESSION 3

Performing the pulley drop movement in a full lunge makes your core muscles work even harder because it increases the level of rotational instability and the stress on your stabilizing muscles. Drop into the lunge position with the pulley machine on your right. Grasping the cable handles, follow the main sequence, keeping your back straight and the core engaged. Carry out the desired number of repetitions on both sides of your body.

Keep your shoulders straight

Push down with your left foot

SINGLE-LEG, SINGLE-ARM CABLE PRESS

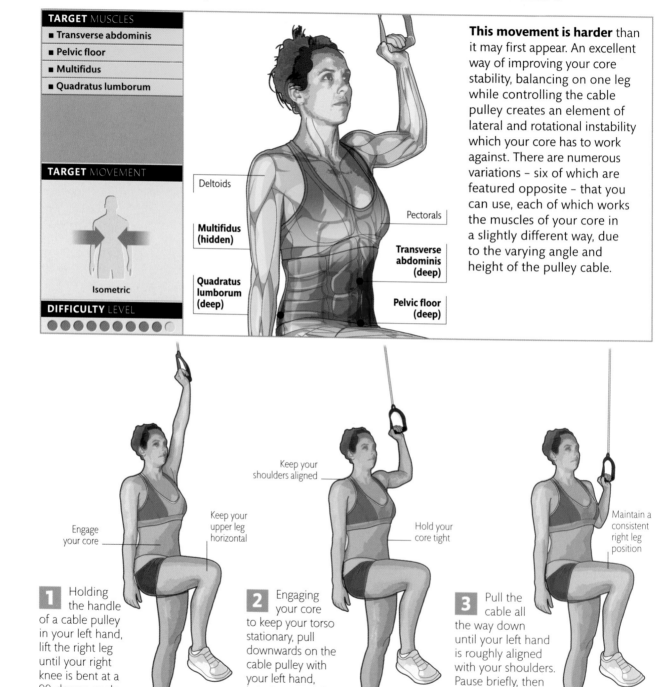

TARGET MUSCLES
- Transverse abdominis
- Pelvic floor
- Multifidus
- Quadratus lumborum

TARGET MOVEMENT

Isometric

DIFFICULTY LEVEL

This movement is harder than it may first appear. An excellent way of improving your core stability, balancing on one leg while controlling the cable pulley creates an element of lateral and rotational instability which your core has to work against. There are numerous variations – six of which are featured opposite – that you can use, each of which works the muscles of your core in a slightly different way, due to the varying angle and height of the pulley cable.

Deltoids

Multifidus (hidden)

Pectorals

Transverse abdominis (deep)

Quadratus lumborum (deep)

Pelvic floor (deep)

1 Holding the handle of a cable pulley in your left hand, lift the right leg until your right knee is bent at a 90-degree angle. Let your right arm hang down by your side.

Engage your core

Keep your upper leg horizontal

2 Engaging your core to keep your torso stationary, pull downwards on the cable pulley with your left hand, bringing your left elbow down towards the body. Keep your back still.

Keep your shoulders aligned

Hold your core tight

3 Pull the cable all the way down until your left hand is roughly aligned with your shoulders. Pause briefly, then return to the start position. Repeat as required, and then switch sides.

Maintain a consistent right leg position

Keep your left foot flat on the floor

VARIATION 1

In this variation of the cable press, carry out the movement in the same position as the basic exercise, but this time place the cable pulley directly in front of you at elbow height. Your left arm should be bent at a 90-degree angle with your upper arm vertical. With your left hand, pull the cable towards you in a horizontal movement. Repeat as required, then switch sides, pulling the cable with your right hand.

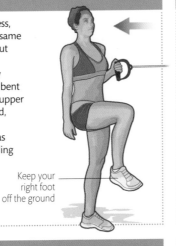

Keep your right foot off the ground

VARIATION 2

This variation is known as a cable row. Begin as normal, but with your left arm lowered and the cable extending upwards from the floor, and not horizontally. Holding the cable pulley in your left hand, carry out the basic movement in reverse, raising your left arm to lift the cable pulley until it is level with your head, with your elbow bent. Lower your arm back down and repeat the exercise as required, before switching sides.

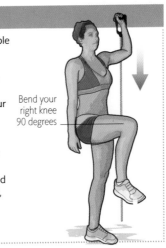

Bend your right knee 90 degrees

VARIATION 3

For this more challenging option, known as the chest fly, run the cable up from the floor as in Variation 2, but this time raise and then lower the cable with your left arm fully extended out sideways from your body, keeping your elbow straight. Keep your right leg lifted, with the knee bent at 90 degrees. Repeat the movement as required, and then switch sides.

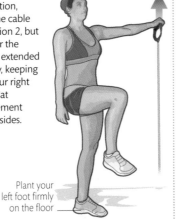

Plant your left foot firmly on the floor

VARIATION 4

In the lateral raise, run the cable horizontally towards you from the left, at shoulder height. Assume the normal start position. With your right knee raised, carry out the movement by pulling the cable pulley across towards your chest until it is level with your left shoulder, and back again. Repeat as required, then switch sides, holding the cable with your right hand and lifting your left knee.

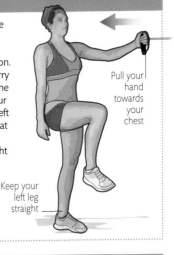

Pull your hand towards your chest

Keep your left leg straight

VARIATION 5

To perform the reverse chop variation of the basic exercise, run the cable pulley towards you from your right side, at head height. Extend your left arm out sideways holding the cable pulley, and raise and bend your right leg to a 90-degree angle. Pull the cable diagonally upwards across your body to the left, keeping your arm straight, then slowly release it and return to the start position. Repeat as required, then switch sides.

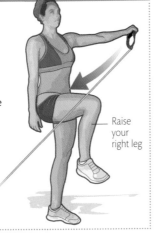

Raise your right leg

VARIATION 6

In this variation, begin with the cable pulley in your right hand. Place the cable in front of you at head height, and to the right. Note that your right leg should be raised at a right angle, as with the left-arm exercises. Extend your right arm sideways, with the elbow slightly bent. Pull the cable straight backwards in a horizontal line, then return to the start position. Repeat as required, then switch sides.

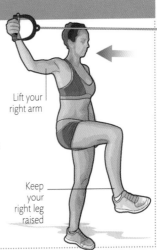

Lift your right arm

Keep your right leg raised

HANGING TOE TUCK

TARGET MUSCLES

- Rectus abdominis
- Transverse abdominis
- Pelvic floor
- Hip flexors
- Gluteus maximus

TARGET MOVEMENT

Flexion

DIFFICULTY LEVEL

This exercise – effectively a more demanding version of the hanging knee-up (»pp.110–11) – may look simple but it is deceptively difficult to perform. Good form is crucial. You must keep your upper body as still and as stable as possible, controlling the movement with your hip flexors and glutes, rather than trying to use momentum.

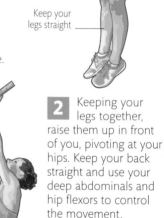

Engage your core

Keep your legs straight

1 Suspend yourself from a chin-up bar with your arms shoulder-width apart, using an underhand grip. Ensure that your legs are straight and stationary, and there is a straight line from your shoulders to your ankle.

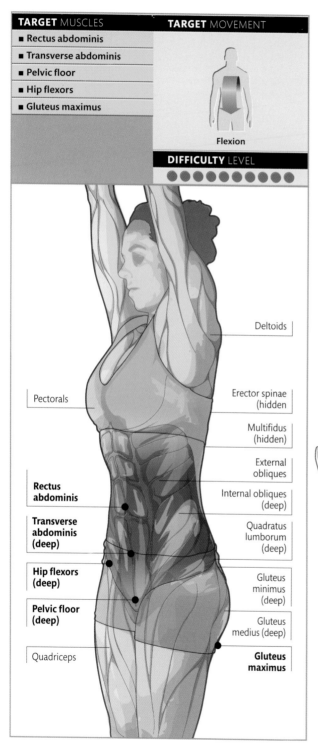

Deltoids

Pectorals

Erector spinae (hidden)

Multifidus (hidden)

External obliques

Rectus abdominis

Internal obliques (deep)

Transverse abdominis (deep)

Quadratus lumborum (deep)

Hip flexors (deep)

Gluteus minimus (deep)

Pelvic floor (deep)

Gluteus medius (deep)

Quadriceps

Gluteus maximus

2 Keeping your legs together, raise them up in front of you, pivoting at your hips. Keep your back straight and use your deep abdominals and hip flexors to control the movement.

Hold your back straight

Keep your knees aligned and together

3 Raise your feet as high as you can manage without straining or compromising your form. Hold briefly, then return to the start position, using your glutes to control the downward movement.

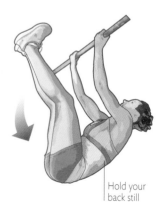

Hold your back still

SANDBAG SHOULDERING

TARGET MUSCLES	TARGET MOVEMENT
■ Transverse abdominis	
■ Internal obliques	
■ Pelvic floor	
■ Erector spinae	
■ Quadratus lumborum	
■ Gluteus maximus	Complex

DIFFICULTY LEVEL

Requiring a combination of core strength and stability, this exercise offers an intensive workout. Good form is key, so focus on perfecting your technique and keeping a straight back throughout before you increase the weight of the sandbag. You should aim to perform the action with a smooth, controlled movement.

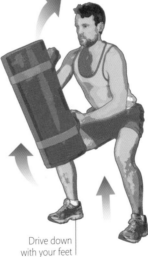

1 Stand with the bag positioned lengthways between your legs. Engage your core, and drop your buttocks backwards into a squat. Grip the handles of the bag, with your right hand to the front.

Straighten your back

Drive down with your feet

2 Driving down with your feet and straightening your legs to stand, lift up the bag vertically in front of you, with your right arm above your left.

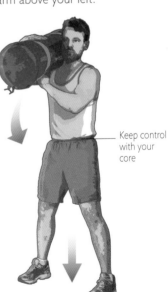

Keep control with your core

3 Continue the movement, lifting the bag on to your right shoulder, letting go of the handle and steadying the bag in the crook of your right arm as you do so. Pause briefly with the bag on your shoulder, then reverse the movement to return to the start position. Repeat as required then switch sides.

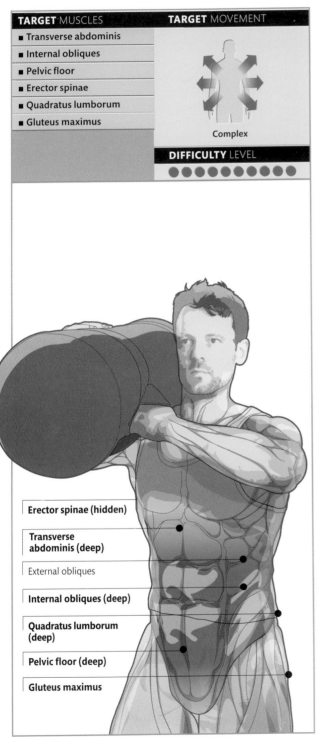

Erector spinae (hidden)

Transverse abdominis (deep)

External obliques

Internal obliques (deep)

Quadratus lumborum (deep)

Pelvic floor (deep)

Gluteus maximus

PLANK PLATE PUSH

TARGET MUSCLES	TARGET MOVEMENT
■ Transverse abdominis	
■ Pelvic floor	
■ Erector spinae	
■ Multifidus	
■ Quadratus lumborum	Isometric

DIFFICULTY LEVEL

This demanding floor exercise combines the basic plank position (**»pp.102–03**) with the dual challenge of moving forwards on your forearms and toes while pushing a weight disc. It offers a superb workout for your core, along with many of the major muscle groups of your upper and lower body. You will need good core strength and a lot of determination to complete the exercise successfully. Because the exercise is tiring, it is very important for you to focus on maintaining good form throughout.

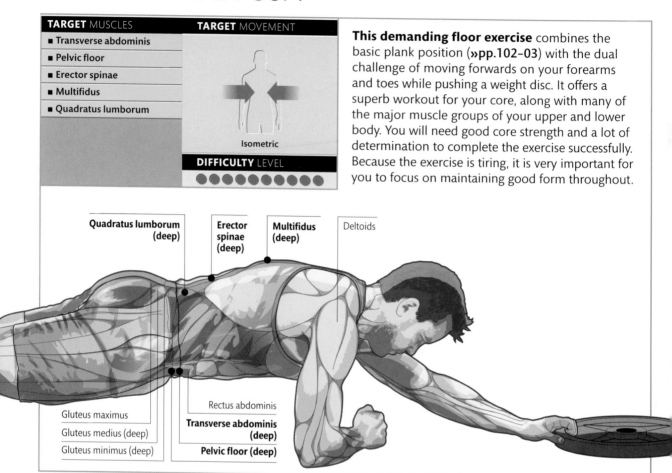

Quadratus lumborum (deep)

Erector spinae (deep)

Multifidus (deep)

Deltoids

Gluteus maximus

Gluteus medius (deep)

Gluteus minimus (deep)

Rectus abdominis

Transverse abdominis (deep)

Pelvic floor (deep)

PROGRESSION

This version of the exercise involves dragging the disc with your feet rather than pushing it in front of you. This makes the movement more challenging because you have to work harder against the force of resistance.

Get yourself into a plank position as before, only this time with the weight disc under your toes. Edge forwards in a regular, crawling movement alternating between each forearm until your feet are extended.

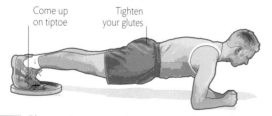

Come up on tiptoe

Tighten your glutes

1 Place a disc on the floor by your feet, and assume a plank position with your toes on the back half of the disc. Use your toes and forearms to support your weight.

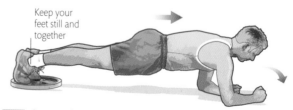

Keep your feet still and together

2 Supporting your weight with your left forearm, drag your body forwards without moving your toes.

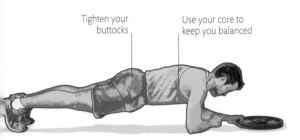

Tighten your buttocks

Use your core to keep you balanced

1 Place a weight disc on the floor in front of you and assume a plank position, with your weight supported on your toes and forearms. Shift your weight to your right forearm and push the disc forwards with your left hand.

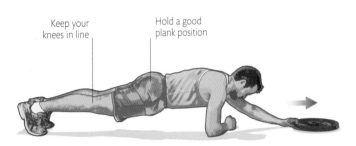

Keep your knees in line

Hold a good plank position

2 Keep pushing the disc until your left arm is fully extended, maintaining the same body position and being careful to keep your core engaged and your glutes tight.

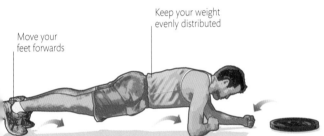

Move your feet forwards

Keep your weight evenly distributed

3 Withdraw your left hand from the disc. Supporting your weight with your left forearm and the toes of your left foot, move your right arm and right leg forwards, maintaining the plank position, and ensuring you keep your back straight.

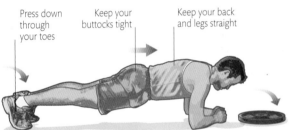

Press down through your toes

Keep your buttocks tight

Keep your back and legs straight

4 Plant your right arm beside your left, and your right foot slightly in front of your left foot, still on your toes. Shifting your weight onto both forearms, bring your left foot forwards and plant it next to your right foot, toes down, as in the start position. Repeat the sequence as required.

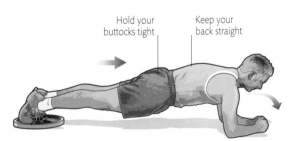

Hold your buttocks tight

Keep your back straight

3 With your weight on your left forearm, bring your right arm forwards to plant it beside your left, keeping your feet still. Your toes should now be extended.

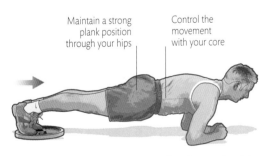

Maintain a strong plank position through your hips

Control the movement with your core

4 Using your core, slide the disc forwards with your toes until you are back in the start position. Repeat the sequence the required number of times.

STEPPED PLANK WALK

TARGET MUSCLES	TARGET MOVEMENT
■ Transverse abdominis	
■ Pelvic floor	
■ Erector spinae	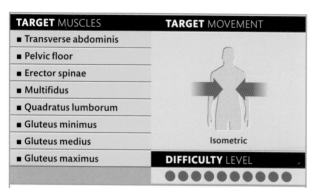
■ Multifidus	
■ Quadratus lumborum	
■ Gluteus minimus	
■ Gluteus medius	Isometric
■ Gluteus maximus	

DIFFICULTY LEVEL
●●●●●●●●●●

This difficult exercise offers a hard full-body workout that requires a lot of practice to perfect. You will need three blocks arranged in shallow steps. Perform the movement in one controlled, fluid motion, and carry out the same number of repetitions for both sides of your body.

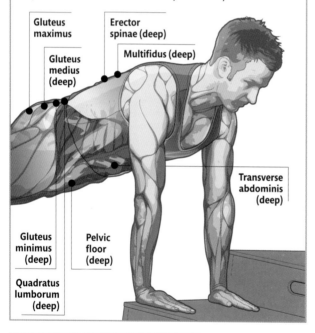

Gluteus maximus

Erector spinae (deep)

Gluteus medius (deep)

Multifidus (deep)

Transverse abdominis (deep)

Gluteus minimus (deep)

Pelvic floor (deep)

Quadratus lumborum (deep)

WARNING!

This exercise requires excellent core stability and is potentially dangerous if performed incorrectly, so only attempt it once you have mastered movements in the earlier sections of the book. Practise without the boxes to begin with, until you are confident in your technique. Always check that the boxes are stable before you begin, and take care when "landing" on the blocks with your hands.

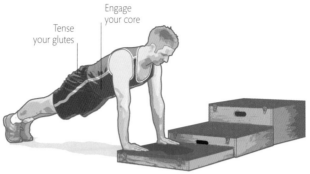

Tense your glutes

Engage your core

1 Begin in the plank position (**»pp.102–03**), with your arms below your shoulders, your hands planted palm-down on the lowest step, your feet together, and your body perpendicular to the blocks.

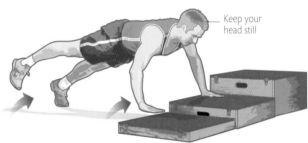

Keep your head still

4 Shifting your weight to your left arm and leg, lift your right hand and leg and move them sideways towards the second step.

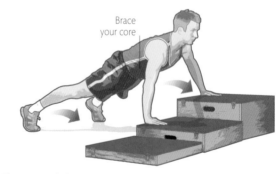

Brace your core

7 Plant your left hand on the third step, and your left foot on the ground, with your right hand still on the second step, and your right foot stationary. Support your weight evenly on both hands and feet.

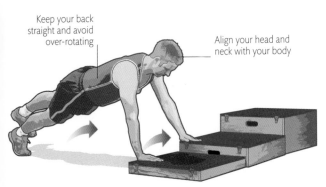

Keep your back straight and avoid over-rotating

Align your head and neck with your body

2 Transferring your weight to your right arm and leg, simultaneously lift your left hand and leg and move them sideways towards the second step.

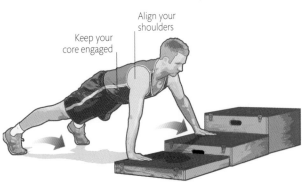

Align your shoulders

Keep your core engaged

3 Plant your left hand on the second step and your left foot on the floor, so that your limbs make a star shape. Support your weight evenly on both sides.

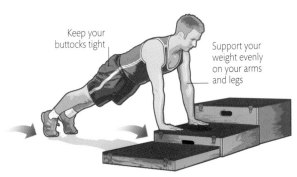

Keep your buttocks tight

Support your weight evenly on your arms and legs

5 Plant your right hand on the second step beside your left, and your right foot beside your left, so that you are in a plank position again.

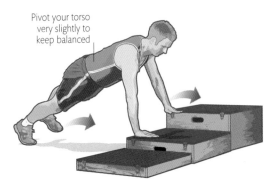

Pivot your torso very slightly to keep balanced

6 As before, transfer the weight to your right arm and leg, and raise your left hand and leg towards the third step, being careful not to over-rotate your body.

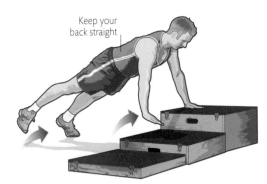

Keep your back straight

8 Shifting your weight to your left arm and leg, as before, raise your right arm and leg and move sideways towards the third step with a smooth, controlled movement.

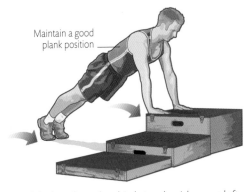

Maintain a good plank position

9 Plant your right hand on the third step beside your left, and your feet together, so that you are back in a plank position. Pause, then reverse the sequence to return to the start. Repeat as required, then switch sides.

TURKISH GET-UP WITH KETTLEBELL

TARGET MUSCLES

- Transverse abdominis
- External obliques
- Internal obliques
- Pelvic floor
- Hip flexors
- Quadratus lumborum
- Gluteus minimus/medius
- Gluteus maximus

TARGET MOVEMENT

Complex

DIFFICULTY LEVEL

This ungainly but highly functional exercise offers an unusual but effective challenge for your core muscles. The basic movement involves raising your body up from a prone position while holding a weight aloft with one hand – in this case a kettlebell. Remember to perform equal numbers of reps with each hand.

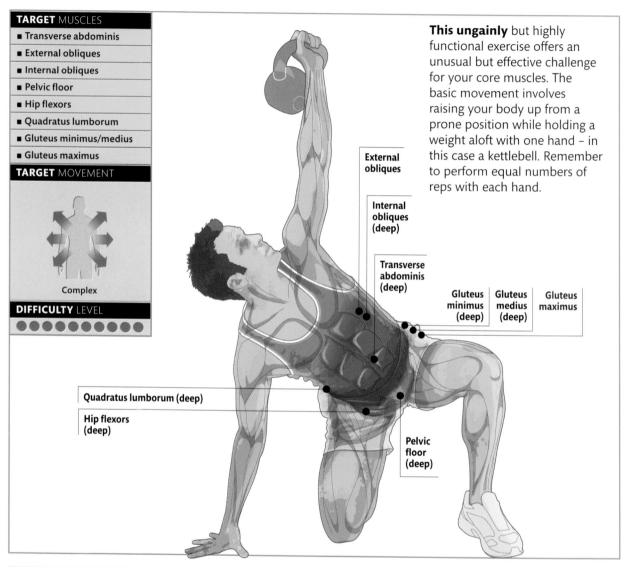

External obliques

Internal obliques (deep)

Transverse abdominis (deep)

Gluteus minimus (deep)

Gluteus medius (deep)

Gluteus maximus

Quadratus lumborum (deep)

Hip flexors (deep)

Pelvic floor (deep)

WARNING!

The Turkish get-up can take a little practice to get right and requires a combination of good core strength and mobility, and flexibility in your joints to perform correctly. With this in mind, it is a good idea to practise and perfect the main part of the movement using the variation (right) to begin with, which will help to reduce the chance of muscle strain or injury as a result of poor form. Because you are holding a weight above your head, make sure you use a light kettlebell to begin with, and always keep a firm grip on the handle.

VARIATION

For a less challenging variation of the Turkish get-up, perform the first three steps of the main exercise (rising to one knee) before returning to the start position, ensuring you carry out the same number of repetitions for both sides. It is also useful for perfecting the key part of the movement.

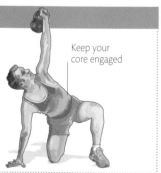

Keep your core engaged

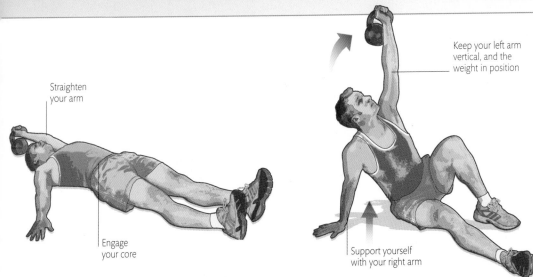

Straighten
your arm

Engage
your core

Keep your left arm
vertical, and the
weight in position

Support yourself
with your right arm

1 Lie on your back and extend your left arm over your head. Grasp a kettlebell with your left hand using an overhand grip and the weight resting against the back of your wrist. Place your right arm at around a 45-degree angle from your body, palm down.

2 Holding your core tight, raise the weight aloft with your left hand and push down with your right hand to lift your upper body off the floor. As you do so, bend your left knee so that you are ready to rise into a kneeling position.

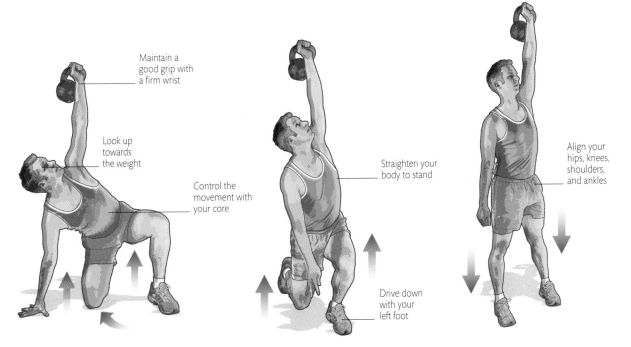

Maintain a
good grip with
a firm wrist

Look up
towards
the weight

Control the
movement with
your core

Straighten your
body to stand

Drive down
with your
left foot

Align your
hips, knees,
shoulders,
and ankles

3 Keeping your core engaged, and the weight held high, push down on your right arm and your left foot, then swing the right leg back and underneath your body.

4 Driving down with your left foot, bring your right arm off the ground and come up on to the toes of your right foot, with your right knee still on the floor.

5 Driving down with both feet, raise yourself to stand, the kettlebell still above your head. Pause, then reverse the movement to return to the start. Repeat as required before switching sides.

EXERCISE BALL HIP ROTATION KICK

TARGET MUSCLES

- Transverse abdominis
- External obliques
- Internal obliques
- Pelvic floor
- Multifidus
- Quadratus lumborum
- Gluteus minimus/medius
- Gluteus maximus

TARGET MOVEMENT

Complex

DIFFICULTY LEVEL

This advanced exercise requires great control, stability, and rotational strength, and offers a challenging workout for all of your core muscles. Do not attempt it unless you have excellent core stability.

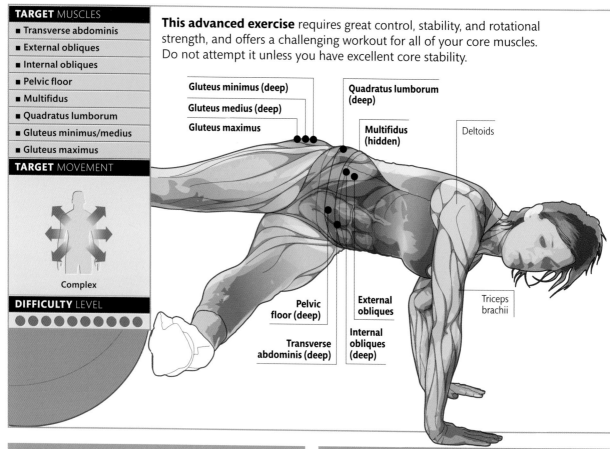

Gluteus minimus (deep)

Gluteus medius (deep)

Gluteus maximus

Quadratus lumborum (deep)

Multifidus (hidden)

Deltoids

Pelvic floor (deep)

External obliques

Transverse abdominis (deep)

Internal obliques (deep)

Triceps brachii

PROGRESSION 1

Performing the exercise with your elbows on an exercise ball increases the instability of the exercise, forcing your core and other muscle groups to work harder. Do not attempt this progression until you have mastered the main exercise.

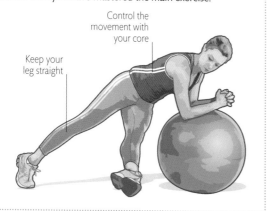

Control the movement with your core

Keep your leg straight

PROGRESSION 2

Carrying out this exercise with your feet on an exercise ball and your hands on a half-exercise ball requires an even greater level of core stability, strength, and flexibility. Do not attempt it until you can perform the less advanced versions with good technique.

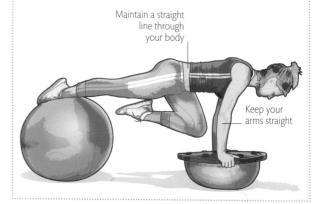

Maintain a straight line through your body

Keep your arms straight

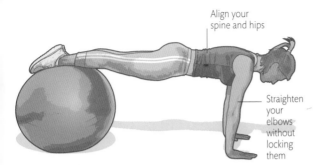

Align your spine and hips

Straighten your elbows without locking them

1 Kneel on the floor with an exercise ball behind you. Place the tops of your feet onto it and, using your core, carefully raise yourself into a press-up position, with your palms flat on the floor.

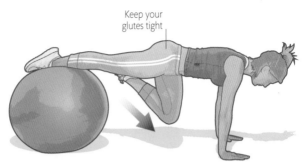

Keep your glutes tight

2 Maintaining a good body position, and with your core engaged, slowly draw your left knee towards your chest until your thigh is at a right angle to your hips.

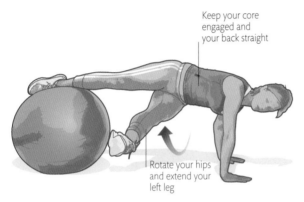

Keep your core engaged and your back straight

Rotate your hips and extend your left leg

3 Pivot your hips to your left and straighten your right knee as you do so, extending your left leg out to your right, bracing yourself with your core.

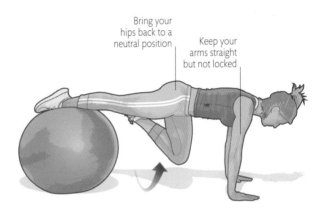

Bring your hips back to a neutral position

Keep your arms straight but not locked

4 Hold briefly, then with control bring your left leg back in and realign your hips, returning to the position shown in Step 2.

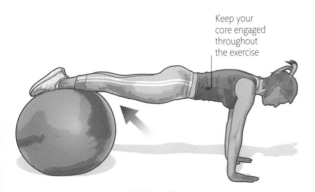

Keep your core engaged throughout the exercise

5 Return to the start position, placing your left foot back on the ball with your knees straight. Repeat the exercise as required, then switch sides.

WARNING!

This exercise requires excellent balance, core control, stability, and mobility to perform. It is important for you to maintain good form throughout the movement. Do not allow your hips or lower back to sag, as this can injure your spine. Use a ball with a diameter that is approximately the length of your arm. This will help you to achieve the correct body position.

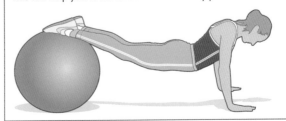

SLIDE BOARD WIPER

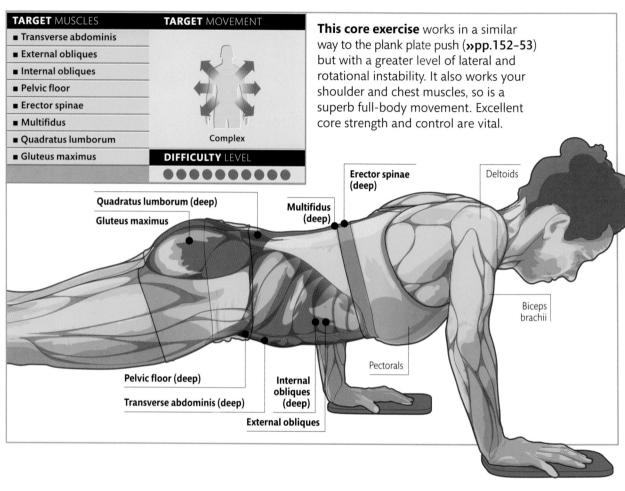

TARGET MUSCLES	TARGET MOVEMENT
■ Transverse abdominis	
■ External obliques	
■ Internal obliques	
■ Pelvic floor	
■ Erector spinae	
■ Multifidus	
■ Quadratus lumborum	Complex
■ Gluteus maximus	**DIFFICULTY** LEVEL

This core exercise works in a similar way to the plank plate push (»pp.152–53) but with a greater level of lateral and rotational instability. It also works your shoulder and chest muscles, so is a superb full-body movement. Excellent core strength and control are vital.

Quadratus lumborum (deep)

Gluteus maximus

Multifidus (deep)

Erector spinae (deep)

Deltoids

Biceps brachii

Pelvic floor (deep)

Transverse abdominis (deep)

Internal obliques (deep)

External obliques

Pectorals

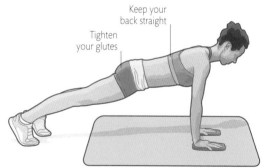

Keep your back straight

Tighten your glutes

1 Position a slide board under each of your hands and begin in the basic plank position. Ensure that you engage your core and hold your glutes tight.

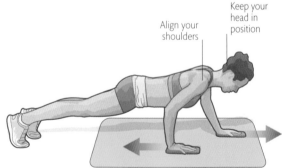

Align your shoulders

Keep your head in position

2 Holding your body in position, simultaneously slide your left hand forwards and your right hand backwards along the floor, bending your elbows slightly as you do so, using your core to balance your weight evenly.

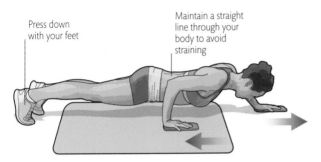

Press down with your feet

Maintain a straight line through your body to avoid straining

3 Continue sliding both hands along the floor, bending your elbows with the movement, until your body is roughly parallel with the floor. Hold briefly at the edge of the movement.

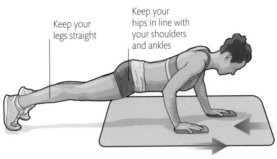

Keep your legs straight

Keep your hips in line with your shoulders and ankles

4 Reverse the movement towards the start position, controlling the movement with your core, and allowing your body to rise.

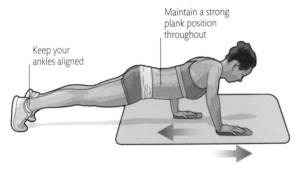

Maintain a strong plank position throughout

Keep your ankles aligned

5 Continue the movement through the start position, sliding forwards with your right hand and backwards with your left hand, controlling the movement with your core and keeping your glutes tight to hold yourself in the plank position.

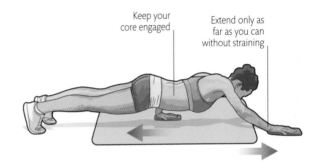

Keep your core engaged

Extend only as far as you can without straining

6 Extend the movement as before, until your body is roughly parallel with the floor, then reverse to begin a return back to the start position, slowly and with good control.

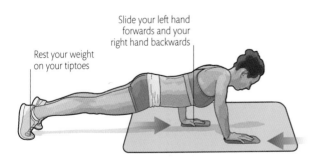

Slide your left hand forwards and your right hand backwards

Rest your weight on your tiptoes

7 Continue the reverse movement, sliding backwards on the slide boards with your right hand and forwards with your left hand. Begin to raise your body up as you bring your hands closer together.

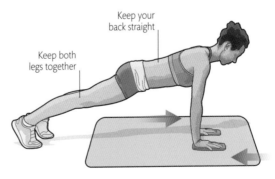

Keep your back straight

Keep both legs together

8 Bring both hands level with your shoulders and return to the start position, raising your body to the press-up position with your core still engaged and your glutes held tight.

RAISED PIKE DUMBBELL HAND-WALK

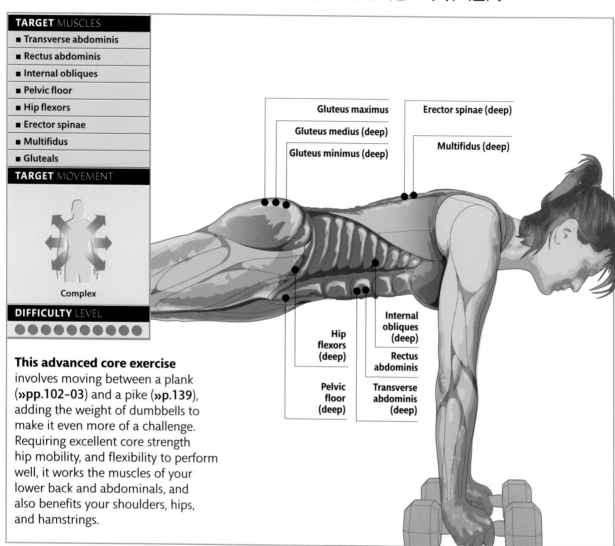

TARGET MUSCLES
- Transverse abdominis
- Rectus abdominis
- Internal obliques
- Pelvic floor
- Hip flexors
- Erector spinae
- Multifidus
- Gluteals

TARGET MOVEMENT

Complex

DIFFICULTY LEVEL

Gluteus maximus

Gluteus medius (deep)

Gluteus minimus (deep)

Erector spinae (deep)

Multifidus (deep)

Hip flexors (deep)

Pelvic floor (deep)

Internal obliques (deep)

Rectus abdominis

Transverse abdominis (deep)

This advanced core exercise involves moving between a plank (»pp.102–03) and a pike (»p.139), adding the weight of dumbbells to make it even more of a challenge. Requiring excellent core strength hip mobility, and flexibility to perform well, it works the muscles of your lower back and abdominals, and also benefits your shoulders, hips, and hamstrings.

WARNING!

You will need a combination of superb flexibility, core strength, and hip mobility to perform this exercise properly. Good technique is crucial because sagging or rounding your back can lead to muscle strain or a more serious back injury, so you should practise and perfect the two basic movements first (»pp.102–03; 139). When assuming the plank position at the start, use your glutes and your core to keep your back straight and avoid your hips or lower back dropping. When moving into the pike position, go only as far as you are able to maintain good form, to avoid the possibility of bending in your lower or mid-back.

PROGRESSION 1

Once you have mastered the basic exercise, you can make it harder by standing on a raised box or stable bench to reduce the support of your legs, making your core work harder to stabilize your body and achieve the pike position.

Engage your core to aid balance

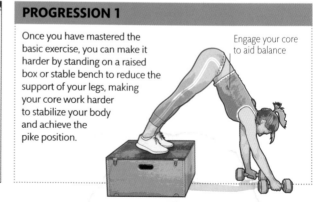

1 Place two dumbbells on the floor in front of you. Grasping a dumbbell in each hand, raise yourself up into a plank position (**»pp.102–03**), holding your core muscles tight and engaging your glutes.

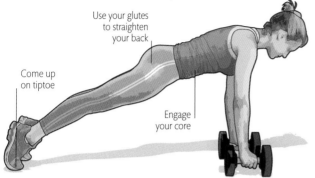

Use your glutes to straighten your back

Come up on tiptoe

Engage your core

2 With a small, smooth movement, "walk" your right hand back towards your feet, shifting the bodyweight on to your left hand as you do so. Keep your legs and back straight, and pivot at your hips.

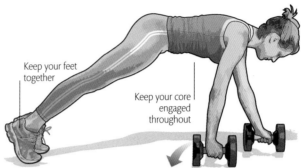

Keep your feet together

Keep your core engaged throughout

3 Plant the dumbbell in your right hand on the floor, then walk your left hand back towards your feet, shifting your bodyweight on to your right hand as you do so, and keeping your legs and back straight. Maintain good form throughout, bending at your hip.

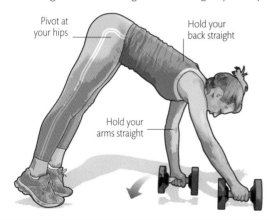

Pivot at your hips

Hold your back straight

Hold your arms straight

4 Plant the dumbbell in your left hand then walk back with your right. Repeat the movement until your back is as close to vertical as you can manage without straining. Hold briefly, then reverse to the start position, slowly and with good form.

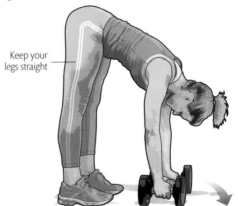

Keep your legs straight

PROGRESSION 2

Raising your feet up on to a half-exercise ball will introduce considerable instability into the basic body position, making your core muscles work much harder to keep you stable. Perform the movement as in the main sequence, focusing on good, controlled form and movement.

Engage your core to aid balance

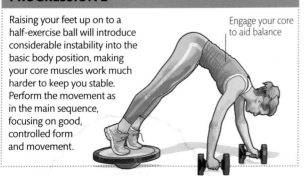

PROGRESSION 3

Performing the movement while extending one leg behind you, requires even greater core stability and hip mobility, as it places additional rotational stress on the muscles of your core. You must have excellent strength and flexibility, so do not attempt it unless you have first mastered the main sequence and the other progressions.

Keep your raised leg in line with your torso

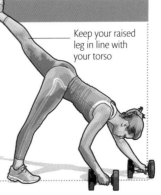

WALL WALK

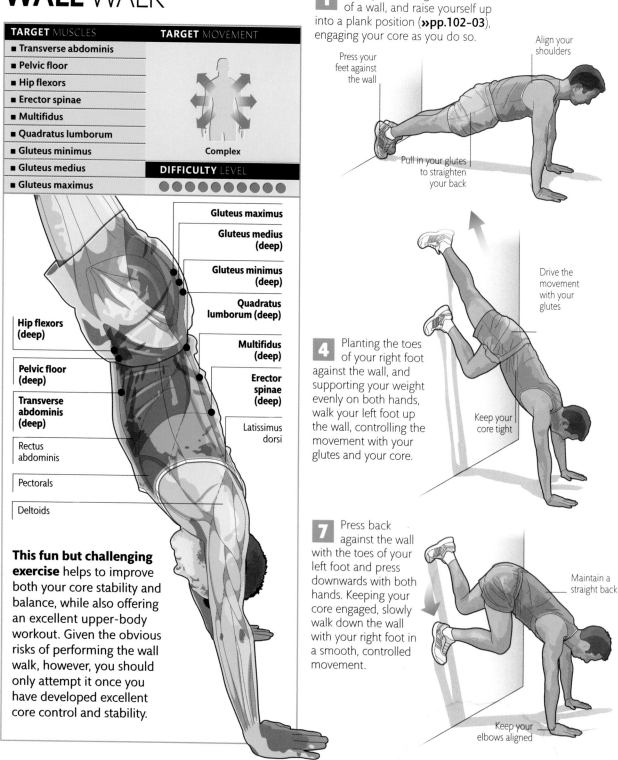

TARGET MUSCLES

- Transverse abdominis
- Pelvic floor
- Hip flexors
- Erector spinae
- Multifidus
- Quadratus lumborum
- Gluteus minimus
- Gluteus medius
- Gluteus maximus

TARGET MOVEMENT

Complex

DIFFICULTY LEVEL

This fun but challenging exercise helps to improve both your core stability and balance, while also offering an excellent upper-body workout. Given the obvious risks of performing the wall walk, however, you should only attempt it once you have developed excellent core control and stability.

Gluteus maximus

Gluteus medius (deep)

Gluteus minimus (deep)

Quadratus lumborum (deep)

Multifidus (deep)

Erector spinae (deep)

Latissimus dorsi

Hip flexors (deep)

Pelvic floor (deep)

Transverse abdominis (deep)

Rectus abdominis

Pectorals

Deltoids

1 Press your feet against the base of a wall, and raise yourself up into a plank position (**»pp.102–03**), engaging your core as you do so.

Align your shoulders

Press your feet against the wall

Pull in your glutes to straighten your back

Drive the movement with your glutes

4 Planting the toes of your right foot against the wall, and supporting your weight evenly on both hands, walk your left foot up the wall, controlling the movement with your glutes and your core.

Keep your core tight

7 Press back against the wall with the toes of your left foot and press downwards with both hands. Keeping your core engaged, slowly walk down the wall with your right foot in a smooth, controlled movement.

Maintain a straight back

Keep your elbows aligned

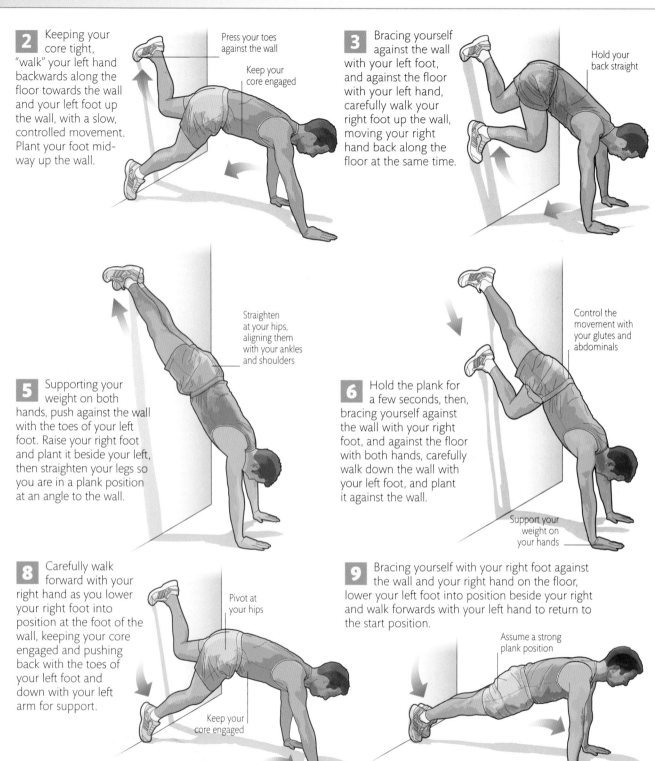

2 Keeping your core tight, "walk" your left hand backwards along the floor towards the wall and your left foot up the wall, with a slow, controlled movement. Plant your foot mid-way up the wall.

Press your toes against the wall

Keep your core engaged

3 Bracing yourself against the wall with your left foot, and against the floor with your left hand, carefully walk your right foot up the wall, moving your right hand back along the floor at the same time.

Hold your back straight

5 Supporting your weight on both hands, push against the wall with the toes of your left foot. Raise your right foot and plant it beside your left, then straighten your legs so you are in a plank position at an angle to the wall.

Straighten at your hips, aligning them with your ankles and shoulders

6 Hold the plank for a few seconds, then, bracing yourself against the wall with your right foot, and against the floor with both hands, carefully walk down the wall with your left foot, and plant it against the wall.

Control the movement with your glutes and abdominals

Support your weight on your hands

8 Carefully walk forward with your right hand as you lower your right foot into position at the foot of the wall, keeping your core engaged and pushing back with the toes of your left foot and down with your left arm for support.

Pivot at your hips

Keep your core engaged

9 Bracing yourself with your right foot against the wall and your right hand on the floor, lower your left foot into position beside your right and walk forwards with your left hand to return to the start position.

Assume a strong plank position

STATIC STRETCHES

Static stretches should always be performed after exercise to help your muscles relax and prevent them becoming shortened, which can lead to injury. Try to combine a range of seated and standing stretches to work a full range of muscles, and ensure you breathe deeply and rhythmically, inhaling before each stretch and exhaling during the movement.

NECK SIDE FLEXION

This static stretch is useful for the muscles of your shoulders and neck. Perform the movement with good control and ensure you repeat it in both directions.

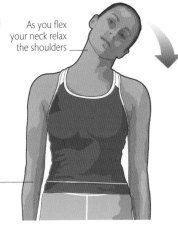

As you flex your neck relax the shoulders

Allow your arms to hang by your sides

Tilt your head towards your left shoulder as far as is comfortable. Hold the stretch briefly, then repeat in the opposite direction.

UPPER-BACK STRETCH

This easy stretch works the muscles in your upper back, making it useful for most sports, but particularly those that involve throwing.

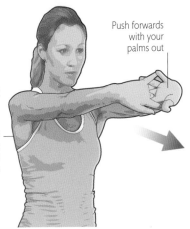

Push forwards with your palms out

Feel the stretch in your upper back and shoulders

Interlocking your fingers, palms facing out, raise your hands up to chest level and extend your arms. Locking out your elbows, push your shoulders forwards. Hold briefly and relax.

PEC STRETCH

This stretch targets the pectoral muscles of your upper chest, easing any tightness and increasing flexibility. It is also helpful if you train for sports that involve throwing.

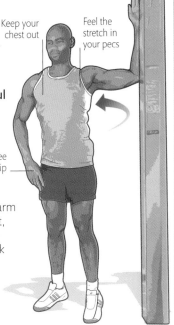

Keep your chest out

Feel the stretch in your pecs

Rest your free hand on your hip

Stand sideways to a solid vertical support. Rest one arm behind the upright support, keeping your upper arm in line with the shoulder. Rock your body gently forwards until you can feel the stretch in your chest. Hold briefly then relax.

LAT STRETCH

Specifically targeting the latissimus dorsi muscles, this stretch is useful for a number of sports, including weightlifting, rowing, and field athletics.

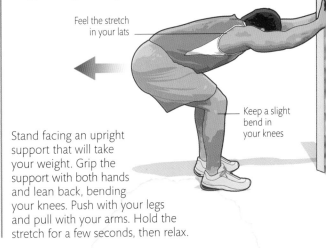

Feel the stretch in your lats

Keep a slight bend in your knees

Stand facing an upright support that will take your weight. Grip the support with both hands and lean back, bending your knees. Push with your legs and pull with your arms. Hold the stretch for a few seconds, then relax.

SEATED TWIST

This exercise works the muscles around your spine and improves the rotational mobility of the upper back. It is important to keep your lower back straight and twist from your shoulders.

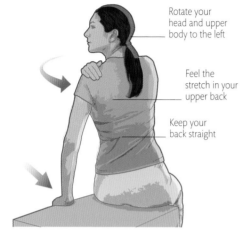

Rotate your head and upper body to the left

Feel the stretch in your upper back

Keep your back straight

Sit on the edge of a box, your feet flat on the floor. Twist to the left, pulling your left shoulder back with your right hand, pushing against the box with your left hand. Hold the stretch briefly, then relax and swap sides.

LATERAL EXTENSION

This is a great stretch for the muscles of your obliques and upper back. Try to lengthen both sides of your upper body as you reach up, and avoid leaning forwards.

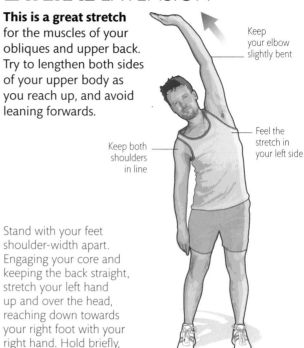

Keep your elbow slightly bent

Feel the stretch in your left side

Keep both shoulders in line

Stand with your feet shoulder-width apart. Engaging your core and keeping the back straight, stretch your left hand up and over the head, reaching down towards your right foot with your right hand. Hold briefly, then switch sides.

STANDING BACK EXTENSION

This simple but effective stretch targets your abdominals, obliques, and hip flexors and helps to improve posture, chest, and neck stiffness.

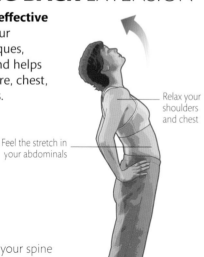

Relax your shoulders and chest

Feel the stretch in your abdominals

Stand upright with your spine in a neutral position and your hands on your hips for support. Raising your chin upwards, extend the back with a slow and controlled movement. Hold the stretch for a few seconds, then relax.

SEATED SPIRAL TWIST

This stretch works your glutes and iliotibial band (ITB), the muscular tissue on the outside of your upper leg. It is important for hip mobility and flexibility, and is especially useful for runners and cyclists.

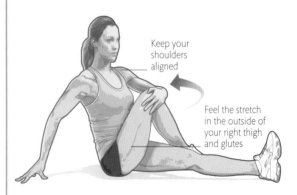

Keep your shoulders aligned

Feel the stretch in the outside of your right thigh and glutes

Sit on the floor with your legs extended and your right hand behind you. Bend your right leg over your left leg and plant your right foot on the floor. Gently press on your right knee with your left hand until you can feel the stretch in the outside of your right leg. Hold briefly, then switch sides.

CAT STRETCH

This static version of the mobility stretch is excellent for working the stabilizing muscles of your spine and lubricating your spinal joints.

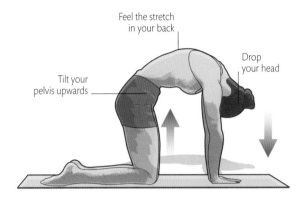

Feel the stretch in your back

Drop your head

Tilt your pelvis upwards

Kneel on all fours with your hands flat on the floor and in line with your shoulders, the fingers forwards, and knees below your hips. Round your back upwards and pull your stomach in, letting your head drop down. Hold briefly, then raise your buttocks and curve your spine down, your head now facing forwards. Hold, then return to the start position.

CHILD'S POSE STRETCH

This movement gently works your spine, hips, thighs, and ankles. Reach forwards with both your hands to maximize the stretch in your back and shoulders.

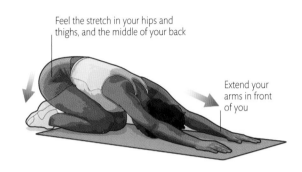

Feel the stretch in your hips and thighs, and the middle of your back

Extend your arms in front of you

Kneel on all fours on a mat with your hands in line with the shoulders, your fingers pointing forwards, and your knees below your hips. Keep your back straight and the head in line with it. With your hands still in position, slowly lower yourself down onto your heels until your forehead touches the mat. Extend your hands forwards to increase the stretch.

HIP FLEXOR STRETCH

This is an excellent static stretch that helps reduce tightness in your hip flexor muscles, which can cause imbalances in your core muscles, and often back pain.

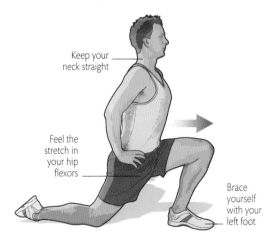

Keep your neck straight

Feel the stretch in your hip flexors

Brace yourself with your left foot

With your hands on your hips, kneel on your right knee, with your left foot in front and your left knee bent at a right angle. Push forwards with your left hip. Hold the stretch, then switch legs.

OBLIQUE STRETCH

This is a good stretch for your internal obliques. Elongate both sides of your torso as you reach up, look straight ahead, and keep your lower back still.

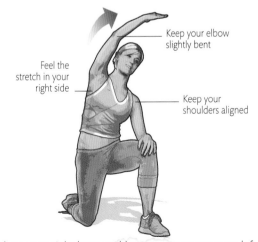

Keep your elbow slightly bent

Feel the stretch in your right side

Keep your shoulders aligned

Kneel on your right knee and lean your torso to your left, pushing your pelvis to the right. Reach across your body with your right arm over your head. Hold briefly, then return to the start.

ABDOMINAL COBRA STRETCH

This is an effective stretch for the stabilizing muscles of the abdominals, obliques, and hip flexors. You should aim to keep your neck and shoulders relaxed throughout in order to avoid straining.

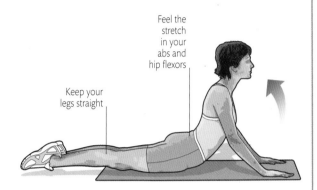

Feel the stretch in your abs and hip flexors

Keep your legs straight

Lie face down on a mat with your hands flat on the floor. Extend your feet, keeping your legs together. Pressing your hips against the mat, raise your torso upwards, using your arms for support. Raise your head and shoulders as high as you can without straining. Hold the stretch for a few seconds and then relax to the start position.

LYING WAIST TWIST

This stretch works the muscles of your lower back and hip joints. Ensure you perform the movement on both sides of your body.

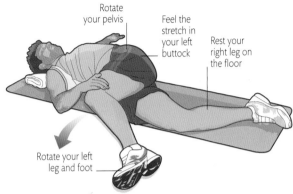

Rotate your pelvis

Feel the stretch in your left buttock

Rest your right leg on the floor

Rotate your left leg and foot

Keeping your upper body flat against the mat, bend your left leg at the knee and bring it across your body, using your right hand to increase the stretch, and allowing your right leg to turn and bend in the same direction. Hold for a few seconds, then switch sides.

HAMSTRING STRETCH 1

It is important to stretch your hamstrings because tightness in the muscles can affect hip mobility and the position of your pelvis, leading to lower back pain. This stretch is useful for lengthening the muscles.

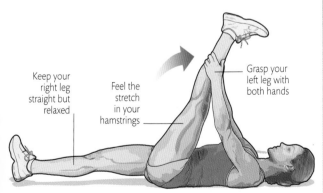

Keep your right leg straight but relaxed

Feel the stretch in your hamstrings

Grasp your left leg with both hands

Lie on your back, and with your right leg extended on the floor, lift your left leg with both hands, keeping your left knee slightly bent and the toes pulled back towards your body. Relax and then repeat the movement with your right leg.

HAMSTRING STRETCH 2

This is a simple general-purpose stretch that works the muscles in your hamstrings, relieving the tightness that can stress your lower back. Stretch slowly and avoid "bouncing" at full extension.

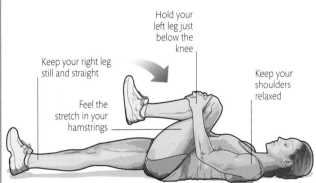

Hold your left leg just below the knee

Keep your right leg still and straight

Feel the stretch in your hamstrings

Keep your shoulders relaxed

Lie on your back with your legs extended. Bend your left knee. Pull gently on your left leg, bringing your knee close to your chest until you feel the stretch. Keep the back of your head on the floor. Relax and repeat with your right leg.

ADDUCTOR STRETCH 1

This stretch works the short adductor muscles of your hips. It is easy to perform but it is important to keep your feet and knees aligned.

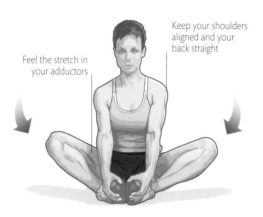

Keep your shoulders aligned and your back straight

Feel the stretch in your adductors

Sit on the floor and grasp the tops of your feet, pressing the soles of them together. Bringing your legs close in towards your body, push down gently with your knees as far as you can, hold for a few seconds, and release.

ADDUCTOR STRETCH 2

This alternative adductor stretch is good for keeping your hips mobile. Avoid stretching down too far and always repeat the stretch on both legs.

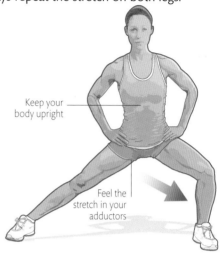

Keep your body upright

Feel the stretch in your adductors

Stand up with your hands on your hips. Bend your left leg so that your left knee is over your left foot, your right leg is extended, and your right foot is flat. Rock gently to the side. Relax and switch legs.

HIP WALK STRETCH

Good hip mobility helps keep your body steady, upright, and well balanced. This simple but effective stretch targets your hips and glutes, and requires good balance. Ensure you perform it on both legs.

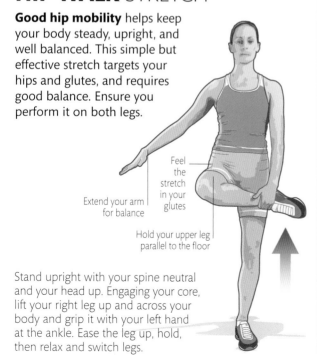

Feel the stretch in your glutes

Extend your arm for balance

Hold your upper leg parallel to the floor

Stand upright with your spine neutral and your head up. Engaging your core, lift your right leg up and across your body and grip it with your left hand at the ankle. Ease the leg up, hold, then relax and switch legs.

ROTATIONAL LUNGE STRETCH

This stretch works your glutes and hip flexors while also promoting good spinal control and stability. Remember to perform it on both sides.

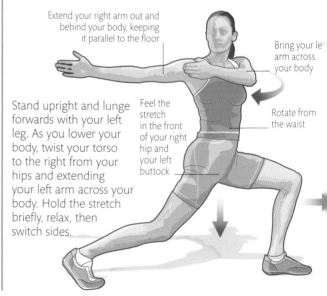

Extend your right arm out and behind your body, keeping it parallel to the floor

Bring your le[ft] arm across your body

Rotate from the waist

Feel the stretch in the front of your right hip and your left buttock

Stand upright and lunge forwards with your left leg. As you lower your body, twist your torso to the right from your hips and extending your left arm across your body. Hold the stretch briefly, relax, then switch sides.

QUAD STRETCH

This stretch works the large quadriceps muscles at the front of your thigh, helping to improve mobility in your hip joints and aiding your posture and balance. Always make sure the table you use is stable enough to take your weight.

Keep your head forwards and your spine neutral

Tilt your pelvis forward slightly

Right leg supports your body

Stand with your back to a steady table. Place your left foot on the table and, keeping your legs parallel, tilt your pelvis forward slightly so you can feel the stretch in the front of your left thigh. Hold, lower your foot, and repeat with your right leg.

ITB STRETCH

This is an excellent stretch for your iliotibial band (ITB), the band of muscle on the outside of your thigh. It helps with hip mobility and flexibility, and can prevent inflammation of the area – iliotibial band syndrome, which is a common cause of pain.

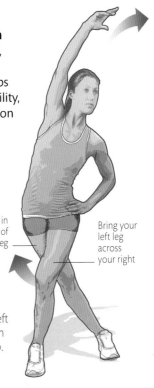

Feel the stretch in the outside of your right leg

Bring your left leg across your right

Stand upright with your feet hip-width apart. Bring your left leg across your right, putting your weight on your left foot, raising your opposite arm above your head as you do so. Hold the stretch briefly, then relax, and switch sides.

STANDING GLUTE STRETCH

This stretch uses a table to work the deep muscles of your gluteals, along with your iliotibial band.

Rest the outside of your left leg on a stable tabletop, bending at your knee, so your right leg is extended and your right foot is up on tiptoe. Tilt your pelvis forwards until you feel the stretch in your left buttock. Hold, relax, and repeat with your right leg.

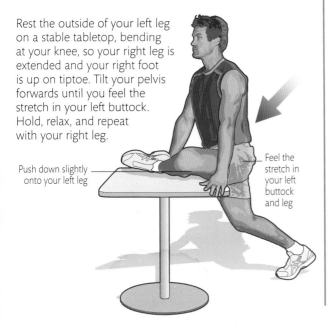

Push down slightly onto your left leg

Feel the stretch in your left buttock and leg

EXERCISE BALL BACK STRETCH

This exercise stretches the joints of your upper and lower back, and helps to improve the alignment of your spinal joints.

Feel the stretch in your upper back and shoulders

Feel the stretch in your abdomen

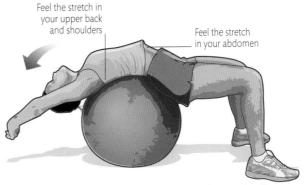

With your feet shoulder-width apart and flat on the floor, squat down onto an exercise ball, and lean back over it so that both your shoulders and buttocks are resting on it. Stretch both arms over your head and allow your arms to fall as far as they will go. Hold the position for a few seconds, breathing in and out, then relax.

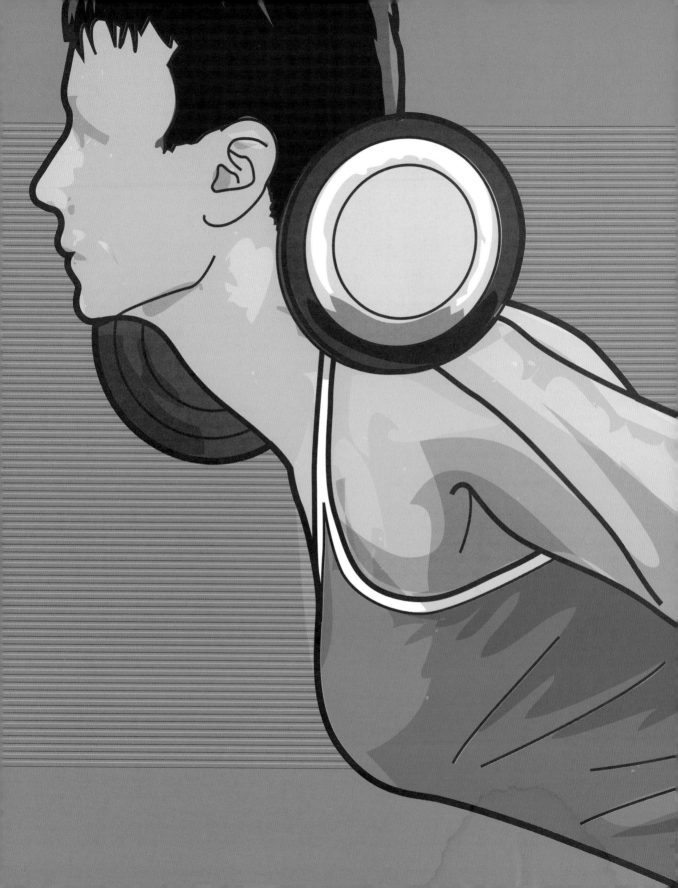

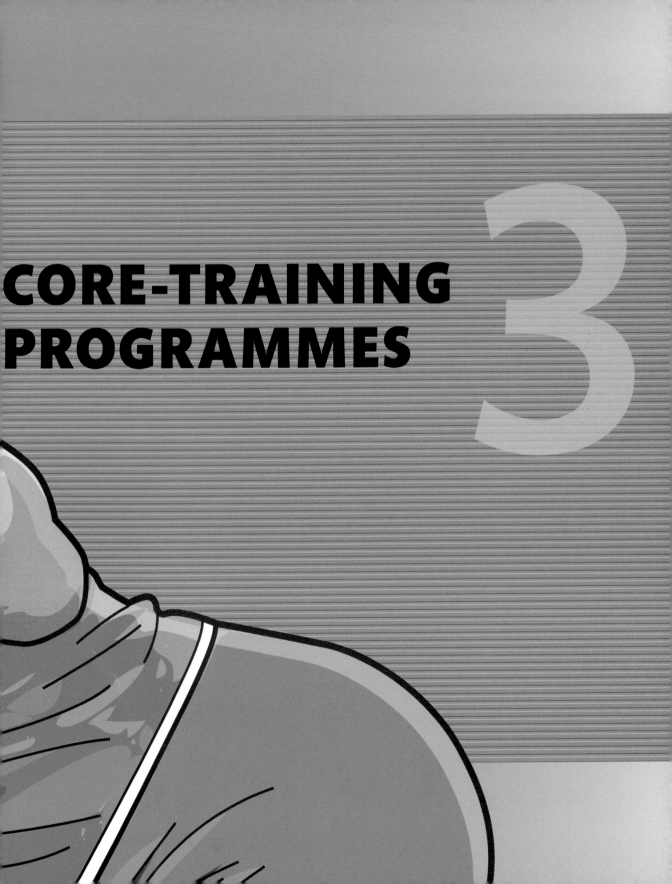

CORE-TRAINING PROGRAMMES

3

INTRODUCTION

The core-training programmes in this section are designed to help you get the very best out of your workouts, whatever your gender, age, experience, or existing level of core strength, stability, and mobility. Using a small number of targeted exercises, each programme will allow you to complete your training session in around 30–40 minutes (the core 300 challenges can be completed as quickly as possible, but remember to maintain good form). All of the featured exercises are covered in more detail in the main exercise section of the book (»pp.42–171).

WARNING!

Before you attempt any of the training programmes in this section, you should also ensure that you have a good base level of core strength: you should be able to achieve a neutral hip position, and to activate your pelvic floor and transverse abdominis muscles (»p.25), and be able to carry out the basic exercises in the Activation and Foundation sections (»pp.56–107). Developing good control of your core muscles and a better understanding of how they work together is vital, as it will give you the best possible results from your training while reducing your risk of injury. Do not be tempted to attempt the more advanced exercises and programmes too soon, as good technique is essential to avoiding injury. If you are carrying, or have recently recovered from an injury, then consult your doctor before you begin (»p.224).

Which programme is right for me?

The first two programmes in this section are designed with the two common core-training goals in mind – developing good overall core strength (»pp.176–77) and improving your posture (»pp.178–79). The third programme is designed specifically for training with bodyweight only (»pp.180–81). The fourth and fifth programmes are designed for training during and after pregnancy (»pp.182–85), with a particular focus on safely targeting the areas of the core most affected by pregnancy. However, before undertaking any form of training while pregnant, you should first seek the advice and guidance of your doctor or equivalent healthcare professional.

BASIC PRINCIPLES

Regardless of the programme you follow, some basic training principles always apply:
- **OVERLOAD:** Your training should demand more of your muscles than would normally be the case for everyday activity.
- **RECOVERY:** An essential component in any training regimen, recovery literally means rest. It is while your body is resting that it adapts and strengthens, preparing to be overloaded again during the next training session.
- **PROGRESSION:** Your body becomes used to the demands being placed on it. If you do not place extra demands on it, your training results will reach a plateau. With this in mind, most of the exercises in the book come with progressions, which you can move on to once you have mastered the main movement.

Each of the example programmes is split into three stages of difficulty, and comes complete with a recommended number of sets and repetitions, recovery times between sets, and suggestions on the ideal duration and frequency of the programmes. This is to help you avoid the risk of overtraining, and enable you to progress your training in a sensible, structured way. You should always begin with the most basic of the programmes, and work your way up to the second and the third as you progress.

The Design Your Own (»pp.186–89) and Challenge 300 (»pp.190–91) programmes pave the way for the next step in training, equipping you with the tools you need to build your own individually tailored programmes, and set yourself challenges and tests to monitor your progress. If you are developing your core strength to meet the needs of a specific sport, you should also refer to the sports-specific section of the book (»pp.192–215) for more information on the primary core movements involved, enabling you to tailor your training programme effectively.

How long should I follow a programme for?

Each of the programmes has a predetermined duration of around 4–14 weeks. If you follow a programme for longer than recommended, your body will adapt to it and plateau, often resulting in a lapse or possible results being be less than expected. Generally speaking, it is advisable to change, progress or even regress your programme every 4–6 weeks. This will help to keep the body challenged and progression consistent, allowing you to gain the most effective results.

Why should I warm up and cool down?

Far too often, warming up and cooling down before and after exercise is a rushed, or completely neglected, part of a training regimen. However, both are essential for getting the best results from training and reducing the risk of injury.

Warming up your muscles before you begin to exercise is essential because it gets your body ready for your workout. Mobilizing your muscles properly gets your joints moving in the correct way, helping you to perform exercises with the best possible form, and reducing the risk of muscular imbalances occuring. Cooling down your muscles after exercise is equally important as it returns your body to a resting state in a controlled manner.

Stretching can be time-consuming, but you should never be tempted to skip your warm-up before your training session or your cool-down at the end of the session. Doing so will increase your risk of injury and hinder your ability to complete your next workout.

How do I warm up and cool down?

For a good basic warm-up, you should begin with 5–10 minutes of light cardiovascular work, such as skipping or jogging, followed by around 10 minutes of dynamic mobility work, ensuring that you work through all of your major muscle groups and joints – see Mobilization for a selection of useful mobility stretches (**»pp.44–55**). You can also tailor your warm-up to your training activity if you need something more specific. A qualified coach or fitness instructor can advise you on this. For a good cool-down session, you should aim to carry out 5–10 minutes of gentle jogging or walking, which decreases both your heart rate and your body temperature, as well as helping your muscles to get rid of any waste products that have built up, such as lactic acid. You should follow this with a further 5–10 minutes of static stretches (**»pp.166–71**) to help your muscles relax and your muscle fibres to re-align and re-establish their

normal resting length and ranges of movement. As for the mobility stretches, aim to work through all of your major muscle groups and joints.

What results should I expect?

If you follow the training programmes properly, you should expect to see results after 4–6 weeks. However, this will vary from person to person, as no two people are exactly the same. There are a range of factors that will affect the speed of your progress:

Age: As well as your age in years, age refers to your emotional and biological maturity as well as the number of years of "training history" you have.

Gender: Men and women have different physiologies and capabilities.

Heredity: This is your innate fitness and ability, which is determined by your genetics.

Physical capability: This is made up of two factors – your heredity and your training history.

Lifestyle: This relates to how well you look after yourself in between training sessions. It can be affected by factors such as diet, rest, and the kind of job you do.

UNDERSTANDING THE CHARTS

These are the terms you need to understand to use the charts effectively and to get the best out of each programme:

■ **MOBILIZATION WARM-UP:** This should be a combination of light cardiovascular work and dynamic stretches (**»pp.44–55**) to activate your core muscles before you begin your training session.

■ **MOVEMENT:** The primary core movement involved in an individual exercise (**»pp.6–7; pp.26–27**) – I = Isometric; F = Flexion; E = Extension; SF = Side Flexion; R = Rotation; C = Complex.

■ **SETS:** A pre-defined group of repetitions separated by a short period of rest – for example, two sets of five repetitions.

■ **REPETITION:** The number of times a weight should be lifted, usually within a single set – "reps" for short.

■ **REST:** The suggested length of the break between individual sets.

■ **MUSCULAR FAILURE:** The point at which you cannot perform another repetition of an exercise within a set.

■ **DURATION OF PROGRAMME:** The range given for the number of weeks a programme should be followed. You should not exceed this number.

■ **FREQUENCY OF PROGRAMME:** The number of workouts you should do per week, with the number of rest days you should take between workouts. You should not exceed this number.

■ **RECOVERY TIME:** The ideal number of days' rest you should take between training sessions.

WARNING!

The programmes in this section have all been designed to provide the correct amount of exercise at the correct level of difficulty to challenge your core without overworking it. You should thus never attempt more than the programmes suggest, as this may cause you to overtrain, which can lead to injury. Always build in time either side of each session to carry out a full warm-up and cool-down, and never attempt to perform a weighted movement with too much weight, or force one if it feels painful.

FUNDAMENTAL CORE

The following three-part programme will help you to build and maintain an excellent level of core strength, stability, and mobility. Each stage provides a structured combination of core movements to ensure a balanced and comprehensive workout.

Whom is it suitable for?

The Fundamental Core programme is designed to be used by anyone who gained a solid base of core mobility, stability, and strength, up to those who are able to perform the exercises in the Intermediate and Advanced sections (**>>pp.108–65**) with good form.

At the very least, you should already have mastered the core activation exercises (**>>p.25**) and worked your way through exercises in the Activation section (**>>pp.56–71**) of the book before you begin the programme.

What are the benefits?

When followed correctly, this complete, three-part programme enables you to progress from Foundation to Advanced level training in 3–4 months, building excellent all-round core strength, stability, and mobility.

How does it progress?

The Foundation stage helps you to build a basic level of core strength, developing your core in all of the planes of movement. The Intermediate programme stage uses exercises that increase the load on your core, making it work harder. The Advanced stage uses extreme exercises that require excellent core mobility, stability, and strength, the majority involving complex core movements.

WARNING!

To avoid the risk of injury you must always complete a stage fully before moving up to the next. Focus on achieving and maintaining good form for each of the exercises you perform, as this is crucial to achieving optimum results. When using weights, you should always start with a light weight and add only 1–2kg (2.2–4.4lb) at a time. If you feel pain, or cannot complete the required number of repetitions with good form and without stopping, you must reduce the weight to prevent causing damage to the muscles. If pain persists, then seek the advice of your doctor.

FOUNDATION (LEVELS 2–4)

Mobilization warm-up (>>pp.44–55) 5–10 mins

EXERCISE	MOVEMENT	PAGE	SETS	REPS	REST (SECS)
Abdominal Crunch	F	72–73	1–2	5–25	30–60
Oblique Crunch	R	79	1–2	2–25 each side	30–60
Dorsal Raise	E	76–77	1–2	5–25	30–60
Bridge	I	98–99	1–2	NMF*	30–60
Heel Reach	SF	82	1–2	5–25 each side	30–60
Reverse Curl	F	75	1–2	5–25	30–60
Super-slow Bicycle	R	95	1–2	5–25	30–60
Dorsal Raise (Prog. 2)	E	76–77	1–2	5–25	30–60
Plank	I	102–03	1–2	NMF*	30–60

* NMF = Near Muscular Failure

Foam roller exercises (>>pp.44–45) and static stretching (>>pp.166–71) 5–10 mins

DURATION OF PROGRAMME
4–6 weeks

FREQUENCY OF PROGRAMME
2–3 workouts per week; 1–2 days' rest between workouts

INTERMEDIATE (LEVELS 4–7)

Mobilization warm-up (>>pp.44–55) 5–10 mins

EXERCISE	MOVEMENT	PAGE	SETS	REPS	REST (SECS)
Partner Ball Swap	F	108–09	2–3	10–30	30–60
Medicine Ball Reverse Throw	E	121	2–3	10–30	30–60
Medicine Ball Slam	F	120	2–3	10–30	30–60
Russian Twist	R	119	2–3	10–30	30–60
Windmill	SF	110–11	2–3	10–30	30–60
Kettlebell Swing	C	129	2–3	10–30	30–60
Standing Plate Twist	R	116	2–3	10–30	30–60
Hanging Knee-up	F	110–11	2–3	10–30	30–60
Exercise Ball Roll-out	I	132–33	2–3	10–30	30–60

Foam roller exercises (>>pp.44–45) and static stretching (>>pp.166–71) 5–10 mins

DURATION OF PROGRAMME
4–6 weeks

FREQUENCY OF PROGRAMME
2–3 workouts per week; 1–2 days' rest between workouts

ADVANCED (LEVELS 8–10)

Mobilization warm-up (>>pp.44–55) 5–10 mins

EXERCISE	MOVEMENT	PAGE	SETS	REPS	REST (SECS)
Pike	F	139	2–4	15–30	30–60
Turkish Get-up with Kettlebell	C	156–57	2–4	5–15 each side	30–60
Exercise Ball Jack-knife	F	142	2–4	10–30	30–60
Exercise Ball Hip Rotation Kick	C	158–59	2–4	10–30 each side	30–60
Stick Crunch	F	140–41	2–4	10–30	30–60
Pulley Chop	R	144–45	2–4	10–30 each side	30–60
Hanging Toe Tuck	F	150	2–4	10–30	30–60
Sandbag Shouldering	C	151	2–4	10–30 each side	30–60
Plank Plate Push	I	152–53	2–4	5–20 metres	30–60

Foam roller exercises (>>pp.44–45) and static stretching (>>pp.166–71) 5–10 mins

DURATION OF PROGRAMME
4–6 weeks

FREQUENCY OF PROGRAMME
2–3 workouts per week; 1–2 days' rest between workouts

GOOD POSTURE

Core training can help to improve posture, rebalancing your muscles, and increasing your overall level of core strength and stability. Your main focus during core training for posture should be to maintain good spinal and hip alignment as you exercise. Good form is key to getting the best results.

Whom is it suitable for?

Postural problems can affect most people at some point in their lives, whether due to the ageing process, over-training, or simply a sedentary lifestyle. This programme is designed with all levels of ability in mind, but you should aim to have practised the core activation exercises (**»p.25**) and Activation (**»pp.56–71**) movements before you begin.

What are the benefits?

This three-part programme will help you to build your core from the inside out, helping you to look and feel better. Working on the deep core muscles first improves your spine and hip stability, helping to relieve tightness in the muscles of your hips, lower back, and shoulders, and strengthen weaknesses in your upper back, abdominals, and pelvic floor.

How do I progress?

This programme is designed to progress very gradually, starting with the Activation and Foundation exercises (**»pp.56–107**), to help connect and strengthen your deep core muscles, before moving on to Intermediate and Advanced exercises (**»pp.108–65**), to develop your core, once you have established good technique and stability.

WARNING!

To avoid the potential risk of injury, follow the programme guidelines carefully, progress through the various stages gradually and focus on good form to establish a strong foundation on which to build your core strength. Do not be tempted to rush through the stages too quickly, as this may be counterproductive, causing tight or over-worked muscles to take over from the smaller, deep, or weaker muscles. If your postural problems are a result of a pre-existing condition you must seek the advice of your doctor first before undertaking the programme.

ACTIVATION (LEVEL 1)

Mobilization warm-up (>>pp.44–55) 5–10 mins

EXERCISE	MOVEMENT	PAGE	SETS	REPS	REST (SECS)
Active Pelvic Floor	I	56–57	1–2	8–10	30–60
Knee Fold	I	60–61	1–2	10–20	30–60
Toe Tap	I	62–63	1–2	10–20	30–60
Prone Abdominal Hollowing	I	64	1–2	8–10	30–60
Dart	E	65	1–2	10–20	30–60
Oyster	I	66	1–2	10–20	30–60
Star	I	68	1–2	10–20	30–60
Back Extension	E	69	1–2	10–20	30–60
Superman	I	70–71	1–2	10–20	30–60

Foam roller exercises (>>pp.44–45) and static stretching (>>pp.166–71) 5–10 mins

DURATION OF PROGRAMME
4–6 weeks

FREQUENCY OF PROGRAMME
2–3 workouts per week; 1–2 days' rest between workouts

FOUNDATION (LEVELS 2–4)

Mobilization warm-up (>>pp.44–55) 5–10 mins

EXERCISE	MOVEMENT	PAGE	SETS	REPS	REST (SECS)
Abdominal Crunch	F	72–73	1–2	10–15	30–60
Leg Circle	I	74	1–2	8–10	30–60
Reverse Curl	F	75	1–2	10–15	30–60
Dorsal Raise	E	76–77	1–2	10–15	30–60
Side Bend	SF	81	1–2	10–15	30–60
Hip Roll	R	88–89	1–2	10–15	30–60
Swim	I	94	1–2	20–30	30–60
Super-slow Bicycle	R	95	1–2	10–20	30–60
Bridge	I	98–99	1–2	10–20	30–60

Foam roller exercises (>>pp.44–45)
and static stretching (>>pp.166–71) 5–10 mins

DURATION OF PROGRAMME
4–6 weeks

FREQUENCY OF PROGRAMME
2–3 workouts per week; 1–2 days' rest between workouts

INTERMEDIATE/ADVANCED (LEVELS 5–10)

Mobilization warm-up (>>pp.44–55) 5–10 mins

EXERCISE	MOVEMENT	PAGE	SETS	REPS	REST (SECS)
Windmill	SF	110–11	1–2	10–15	30–60
Exercise Ball Abdominal Crunch	F	73 (Prog.3)	1–2	10–15	30–60
Kettlebell Round-body Swing	I	117	1–2	10–15	30–60
Exercise Ball Back Extension	E	122	1–2	10–15	30–60
Core Board Rotation	I	131	2–4	10–15	30–60
Suspended Crunch	F	134	1–2	8–10	30–60
Exercise Ball Jackknife	I	142	1–2	10–15	30–60
Pulley Chop	R	144–45	1–2	8–10	30–60
Pulley Lift	R	146–47	1–2	10–15	30–60

Foam roller exercises (>>pp.44–45)
and static stretching (>>pp.166–71) 5–10 mins

DURATION OF PROGRAMME
4–6 weeks

FREQUENCY OF PROGRAMME
2–3 workouts per week; 1–2 days' rest between workouts

BODYWEIGHT CORE TRAINING

Bodyweight training can be used for an easy, effective, and versatile core workout. The following programme is designed to be performed anywhere and with the bare minimum of equipment, making it useful if you want to exercise at home.

Whom is it suitable for?

This three-part programme is designed for anyone with a solid base of core mobility, stability, and strength, who is looking for a workout they can use outside the gym, which requires the minimum of equipment. At the very least you should already be able to activate your core (**»p.25**) and perform all of the exercises in the Activation section (**»pp.56–71**) with good form before you begin.

What are the benefits?

The programme is designed to strengthen your core in a balanced way, encouraging a full-body approach. Many of the bodyweight exercises (such as the plank) focus on isometric core stability, which is great for strengthening the upper and lower body as well as the core.

How will I progress?

Even if you train regularly, you should begin with the Foundation stage of the programme, in order to develop a good understanding of your natural range of mobility and core stability, before you move on to the more challenging exercises of the intermediate and advanced progamme stages, which require greater strength and control. Once you have mastered each of the three stages you can try swapping individual exercises with others of a similar movement and difficulty (**»pp.40–43**).

WARNING!

Attention to range of movement, spine and hip alignment, and good all-round technique are vital to achieve the best results and avoid the risk of injury. Practise and progress gradually through the stages to achieve optimum results and avoid over-training. If you feel discomfort or pain, or cannot complete the required number of repetitions with good form and without stopping, you must reduce the weight to prevent causing damage to the muscles. If pain persists, then seek the advice of your doctor.

FOUNDATION (LEVELS 2–4)					
Mobilization warm-up (>>pp.44–55) 5–10 mins					
EXERCISE	MOVEMENT	PAGE	SETS	REPS	REST (SECS)
Abdominal Crunch	F	72–73	1–2	10–15	30–60
Reverse Curl	F	75	1–2	10–15	30–60
Dorsal Raise	E	76–77	1–2	10–15	30–60
Side-lying Lateral Crunch	LF	80	1–2	10–15	30–60
Side-lying Leg Lift	I	84–85	1–2	10–15	30–60
Hip Roll	R	88–89	1–2	10–15	30–60
Roll-up	F	91	1–2	6–10	30–60
Swim	I	94	1–2	20–30	30–60
Side Plank	I	104–05	1–2	6–10	30–60
Foam roller exercises (>>pp.44–45) and static stretching (>>pp.166–71) 5–10 mins					

DURATION OF PROGRAMME
4–6 weeks

FREQUENCY OF PROGRAMME
2–3 workouts per week; 1–2 days' rest between workouts

INTERMEDIATE (LEVELS 5-7)

Mobilization warm-up (>>**pp.44-55**) 5-10 mins

EXERCISE	MOVEMENT	PAGE	SETS	REPS	REST (SECS)
Exercise Ball Abdominal Crunch	F	73 (Prog.3)	1-2	10-15	30-60
Hanging Knee-up	F	110-11	1-2	6-10	30-60
Mountain Climber	I	118	1-2	20-40	30-60
Exercise Ball Back Extension	E	122	1-2	10-15	30-60
Suspended Pendulum	C	127	1-2	6-10	30-60
Suspended Single-arm Core Rotation	R	126	1-2	6-10	30-60
Exercise Ball Roll-out	C	132-33	1-2	10-15	30-60
Suspended Crunch	C	134	1-2	6-10	30-60
Suspended Oblique Crunch	C	135	1-2	6-10	30-60

Foam roller exercises (>>**pp.44-45**)
and static stretching (>>**pp.166-71**) 5-10 mins

DURATION OF PROGRAMME
4-6 weeks

FREQUENCY OF PROGRAMME
2-3 workouts per week; 1-2 days' rest between workouts

ADVANCED (LEVELS 6-10)

Mobilization warm-up (>>**pp.44-55**) 5-10 mins

EXERCISE	MOVEMENT	PAGE	SETS	REPS	REST (SECS)
Exercise Ball Jackknife	F	142	1-2	10-15	30-60
Pike	F	139	1-2	6-10	30-60
Stick Crunch	F	140-41	1-2	6-10	30-60
Wall Walk	I	164-65	1-2	6-10	30-60
Exercise Ball Back Extension	E	122	1-2	10-15	30-60
Hanging Toe Tuck	F	150	1-2	6-10	30-60
Stepped Plank Walk	I	154-55	1-2	6-10	30-60
Exercise Ball Hip Rotation Kick	C	158-59	1-2	6-10	30-60
Slide Board Wiper	C	160-61	1-2	10-15	30-60

Foam roller exercises (>>**pp.44-45**)
and static stretching (>>**pp.166-71**) 5-10 mins

DURATION OF PROGRAMME
4-6 weeks

FREQUENCY OF PROGRAMME
2-3 workouts per week; 1-2 days' rest between workouts

CORE TRAINING FOR PREGNANCY

Core training can be useful for expectant mothers and have a positive effect on overall wellbeing. This three-stage programme is designed to build core mobility, stability, and strength safely to help your body adjust to the physical, postural, and hormonal changes that occur during pregnancy.

Whom is it suitable for?

This programme is suitable for anyone wishing to start or continue with their core training during pregnancy. Each stage addresses the changes that occur in that respective trimester, making the programme safe and effective, without compromising the health or comfort of the mother or baby.

What are the benefits?

Combining a range of core-activation exercises with static stretches, this programme will help to activate your pelvic floor and the deep core muscles of your abdominals and back, helping to relieve back tension and increase lumbar and hip stability. It will also strengthen your core to support the extra weight and aid your balance as your baby grows.

How will I progress?

Due to the changes in weight, shape, size, and balance that occur to the body during the stages of pregnancy, you should limit your training programmes to gentle static stretches and exercises in the book's Activation section (>>pp.56–71), and adhere closely to the structure of the programme.

WARNING!

During pregnancy, you must seek the advice and guidance of your doctor and/or midwife before and during any form of core-strength programme. The overall aim of training during pregnancy is to support the health and wellbeing of both mother and baby and to avoid increasing the stress on your body. With that in mind, you should stick to the programme, taking care not to overtrain or place any additional stress on your body by attempting exercises of a higher level. As you enter your second trimester, you should avoid lying supine for prolonged periods of time because compression on the vena cava may reduce blood flow to the placenta, resulting in supine hypotensive syndrome.

FIRST TRIMESTER (0–12 WEEKS)

Mobilization warm-up (>>pp.44–55) 5–10 mins

EXERCISE	MOVEMENT	PAGE	SETS	REPS	REST (SECS)
Active Pelvic Floor	I	56–57	1–2	5–10	30–60
Knee Fold	I	60–61	1–2	5–10	30–60
Toe Tap	I	62–63	1–2	5–10	30–60
Prone Abdominal Hollowing	I	64	1–2	5–10	30–60
Dart	E	65	1–2	5–10	30–60
Prone Leg Lift	I	67	1–2	5–10	30–60
Star	I	68	1–2	5–10	30–60
Back Extension	I	69	1–2	5–10	30–60
Bridge	I	98–99	1–2	5–10	30–60

Foam roller exercises (>>pp.44–45) and static stretching (>>pp.166–71) 5–10 mins

DURATION OF PROGRAMME
12 weeks

FREQUENCY OF PROGRAMME
2–3 workouts per week; 1–2 days' rest between workouts

SECOND TRIMESTER (13–26 WEEKS)

Mobilization warm-up (>>**pp.44–55**) 5–10 mins

EXERCISE	MOVEMENT	PAGE	SETS	REPS	REST (SECS)
Active Pelvic Floor	I	56–57	1–2	5–10	30–60
Pillow Squeeze	I	58	1–2	5–10	30–60
Heel Slide	I	59	1–2	5–10	30–60
Knee Fold	I	60–61	1–2	5–10	30–60
Oyster	I	66	1–2	5–10	30–60
Superman	I	70–71	1–2	5–10	30–60
Horizontal Balance	I	97	1–2	5–10	30–60
Bridge	I	98–99	1–2	5–10	30–60
Child's Pose Stretch	Stretch	168	1–2	5–10	30–60

Foam roller exercises (>>**pp.44–45**)
and static stretching (>>**pp.166–71**) 5–10 mins

DURATION OF PROGRAMME
13 weeks

FREQUENCY OF PROGRAMME
2–3 workouts per week; 1–2 days' rest between workouts

THIRD TRIMESTER (27–40 WEEKS)

Mobilization warm-up (>>**pp.44–55**) 5–10 mins

EXERCISE	MOVEMENT	PAGE	SETS	REPS	REST (SECS)
Active Pelvic Floor	I	56–57	1–2	5–10	30–60
Pillow Squeeze	I	58	1–2	5–10	30–60
Heel Slide	I	59	1–2	5–10	30–60
Oyster	I	66	1–2	5–10	30–60
Superman	I	70–71	1–2	5–10	30–60
Horizontal Balance	I	97	1–2	5–10	30–60
Bridge	I	98–99	1–2	5–10	30–60
Cat Stretch	Stretch	168	1–2	5–10	30–60
Child's Pose Stretch	Stretch	168	1–2	5–10	30–60

Foam roller exercises (>>**pp.44–45**)
and static stretching (>>**pp.166–71**) 5–10 mins

DURATION OF PROGRAMME
14 weeks

FREQUENCY OF PROGRAMME
2–3 workouts per week; 1–2 days' rest between workouts

POST-PREGNANCY CORE TRAINING

Reduced activity during pregancy, the over-stretching of muscles during childbirth, and the various other physical and hormonal changes that occur to your body can all affect your core strength. This three-stage programme is designed to help you rebuild your core strength safely and gradually.

Whom is it suitable for?

This programme is suitable for all new mothers, providing they have the consent of their doctor and/or midwife before beginning. General exercise is not recommended for the first six weeks following birth, so the first stage of the programme comprises Activation exercises (**»pp.56–71**) only, to ensure you work safely and effectively during this period.

What are the benefits?

Months of inactivity and over-stretched muscles will weaken the abdominals, leaving new mothers prone to back pain and injury as well as loss of balance and core control. The programme will help strengthen your pelvic floor and deep core muscles, increasing the stability and strength of your abdominals, back, and hip muscles, improving posture and balance, and relieving back pain and tension.

How will I progress?

It is important to follow the programme properly and take your training slowly and gradually. The body goes through a huge number of changes before and after birth so will need time and attention in restoring strength. Do not be tempted to rush through the programmes, as this can be counterproductive and may cause complications.

WARNING!

Always seek the approval of your doctor and/or midwife before you start any form of training programme post-pregnancy, and take particular care if you have had a Caesarean birth. Diastasis recti (the separation of the abdominals) is a common concern with regards to core-strength training post-pregnancy, so you should avoid exercises involving spinal flexion until after the separation has decreased. The hormone relaxin will still be at high levels for up to six months after giving birth, so avoid over-stretching and focus on core stability exercises instead.

0–6 WEEKS					
Mobilization warm-up (>>pp.44–55) 5–10 mins					
EXERCISE	MOVEMENT	PAGE	SETS	REPS	REST (SECS)
Active Pelvic Floor	I	56–57	1–2	5–10	30–60
Pillow Squeeze	I	58	1–2	5–10	30–60
Heel Slide	I	59	1–2	5–10	30–60
Prone Abdominal Hollowing	I	64	1–2	5–10	30–60
Dart	E	65	1–2	5–10	30–60
Oyster	I	66	1–2	5–10	30–60
Prone Leg Lift	I	67	1–2	5–10	30–60
Superman	I	70–71	1–2	5–10	30–60
Bridge	I	98–99	1–2	5–10	30–60
Foam roller exercises (>>pp.44–45) and static stretching (>>pp.166–71) 5–10 mins					

DURATION OF PROGRAMME
6 weeks

FREQUENCY OF PROGRAMME
2–3 workouts per week; 1–2 days' rest between workouts

6–12 WEEKS					
Mobilization warm-up (>>pp.44–55) 5–10 mins					
EXERCISE	MOVEMENT	PAGE	SETS	REPS	REST (SECS)
Active Pelvic Floor	I	56–57	1–2	5–10	30–60
Knee Fold	I	60–61	1–2	5–10	30–60
Prone Abdominal Hollowing	I	64	1–2	5–10	30–60
Star	I	68	1–2	5–10	30–60
Leg Circle	I	74	1–2	5–10	30–60
Dorsal Raise	E	76–77	1–2	5–10	30–60
Side-lying Leg Lift	I	84–85	1–2	5–10	30–60
Bridge	I	98–99	1–2	5–10	30–60
Plank	I	102–03	1–2	5–10	30–60
Foam roller exercises (>>pp.44–45) and static stretching (>>pp.166–71) 5–10 mins					

DURATION OF PROGRAMME
6 weeks

FREQUENCY OF PROGRAMME
2–3 workouts per week; 1–2 days' rest between workouts

12 WEEKS ONWARDS					
Mobilization warm-up (>>pp.44–55) 5–10 mins					
EXERCISE	MOVEMENT	PAGE	SETS	REPS	REST (SECS)
Knee Fold	I	60–61	1–2	5–10	30–60
Toe Tap	I	62–63	1–2	5–10	30–60
Oyster	I	66	1–2	5–10	30–60
Abdominal Crunch	F	72–73	1–2	5–10	30–60
Heel Reach	SF	82	1–2	5–10	30–60
Hip Roll	R	88–89	1–2	5–10	30–60
Swim	I	94	1–2	5–10	30–60
Side Plank	I	104–05	1–2	5–10	30–60
Single-leg Extension and Stretch	I	106	1–2	5–10	30–60
Foam roller exercises (>>pp.44–45) and static stretching (>>pp.166–71) 5–10 mins					

DURATION OF PROGRAMME
6 weeks +.

FREQUENCY OF PROGRAMME
2–3 workouts per week; 1–2 days' rest between workouts

DESIGN YOUR OWN (LEVELS 1-4)

The following table offers an easy way to build your core-training programme using a selection of exercises from the Activation and Foundation sections (**»pp.56–107**) offering a balance of core movements. Before you begin designing your own workouts you should first have mastered exercises in the Activation section (**»pp.56–71**) and tried one or two of the other programmes in this chapter.

Whom is it suitable for?

The flexibility of this programme makes it suitable for all levels of ability. Being able to choose the exercises yourself means you can tailor your training to suit your specific needs. However, you should be able to activate your core (**»p.25**) and have worked your way through exercises in the Activation section before you begin.

What are the benefits?

This programme will help you to build a strong, stable, and mobile core, because it trains your muscles across all of the core training movements. Being in control of your own programme is also a great way of ensuring you progress at the right speed for you. Selecting your own exercises and moving onto harder ones when the time is right helps you to develop your core strength correctly and safely, keeping you highly motivated and reducing your risk of over-training, injury, and frustration.

How will I progress?

To begin with you should aim to work through each of the movement patterns level by level, beginning with Level 1, ensuring that you are able to complete a high number of reps and sets – usually 2–3 sets of 20–30 reps – with good technique before you move on to the next level. Conversely, if you feel that an exercise is too difficult, you can replace it with an alternative with the same movement pattern that is one level below. Once you can perform all of the exercises with good form, you can then mix and match, you can then move on to the next Design Your Own programme (**»pp.188–89**) which use exercises from the Intermediate and Advanced sections (**»pp.108–65**) of the book.

Mobilization warm-up (**»pp.44–55**) 5–10 mins					
EXERCISE	**LEVEL**	**PAGE**	**SETS**	**REPS**	**REST (SECS)**
1. ISOMETRIC EXERCISES (CHOOSE ONE...)					
Active Pelvic Floor	1	56–57	2–3	10–12	30–60
Leg Circle	2	74	2–3	10–12	30–60
Swim	3	94	2–3	10–12	30–60
Horizontal Balance	4	97	2–3	10–12	30–60
4. ISOMETRIC EXERCISES (CHOOSE ONE...)					
Heel Slide	1	59	2–3	10–12	30–60
Side-lying Leg Lift	2	84-85	2–3	10–12	30–60
Swim	3	94	2–3	10–12	30–60
Plank	4	102-03	2–3	10–12	30–60
7. FLEXION EXERCISES (CHOOSE ONE...)					
Sit-up	2	78	2–3	10–12	30–60
Roll-up	3	91	2–3	10–12	30–60
V Sit-up	3	93	2–3	10–12	30–60
Double-leg Extension and Stretch	4	107	2–3	10–12	30–60

"DESIGN YOUR OWN" PROGRAMME (LEVELS 1-4)

EXERCISE	LEVEL	PAGE	SETS	REPS	REST (SECS)
2. FLEXION EXERCISES (CHOOSE ONE...)					
Abdominal Crunch	2	72-73	2-3	10-12	30-60
Reverse Curl	2	75	2-3	10-12	30-60
V Leg-raise	3	92	2-3	10-12	30-60
Single-leg Extension and Stretch	4	106	2-3	10-12	30-60
5. SIDE FLEXION EXERCISES (CHOOSE ONE...)					
Side-lying Lateral Crunch	2	80	2-3	10-12	30-60
Side Bend	2	81	2-3	10-12	30-60
Heel Reach	2	82	2-3	10-12	30-60
Roman Chair Side Bend	2	83	2-3	10-12	30-60
8. ISOMETRIC EXERCISES (CHOOSE ONE...)					
Knee Fold	1	60-61	2-3	10-12	30-60
Leg Circle	2	74	2-3	10-12	30-60
Double-leg Lower and Lift	4	100-01	2-3	10-12	30-60
Side Plank	3	104-05	2-3	10-12	30-60

EXERCISE	LEVEL	PAGE	SETS	REPS	REST (SECS)
3. EXTENSION EXERCISES (CHOOSE ONE...)					
Dart	1	65	2-3	10-12	30-60
Back Extension	1	69	2-3	10-12	30-60
Dorsal Raise	2	76-77	2-3	10-12	30-60
Dorsal Raise (Prog. 2)	3	76-77	2-3	10-12	30-60
6. ROTATION EXERCISES (CHOOSE ONE...)					
Oblique Crunch	2	79	2-3	10-12	30-60
Oblique Reach	2	86-87	2-3	10-12	30-60
Hip Roll	2	88-89	2-3	10-12	30-60
Super-slow Bicycle	3	95	2-3	10-12	30-60

Foam roller exercises (**»pp.44–45**)
and static stretching (**»pp.166–71**) 5-10 mins

DURATION
4-6 weeks

FREQUENCY
2-3 workouts per week; 1-2 days' rest between workouts

DESIGN YOUR OWN (LEVELS 5–10)

The table opposite works in the same way as the Design Your Own (Levels 1–4) programme (**»pp.186–87**), except it draws on a more challenging range of exercises from the Intermediate and Advanced sections (**»pp.108–65**). Before you begin you should have a very good level of core strength, stability, and mobility, and you should be able to perform a range of Intermediate and Advanced exercises with good form.

Whom is it suitable for?

The flexibility of this programme makes it suitable for people who have completed the equivalent programme for levels 1–4 (**»pp.186–87**) and are able to carry out most of the exercises in the Intermediate and Advanced sections with good technique.

What are the benefits?

Because it trains your core across all six core movements this programme will help you to build a strong, stable, and mobile core. Designing your own programme enables you to progress at your own speed, developing your core strength in a safe and structured way, to reduce the risk of overtraining, while keeping you fully motivated.

How will I progress?

Before you begin, you should already have completed the three stages of the easier Design Your Own programme, and be able to carry out the exercises featured here with good form. Aim to work through each of the movement patterns level by level, beginning with Level 5, making sure that you can complete a high number of repetitions and sets of the exercise – usually 2–3 sets of 20–30 reps – before moving up to the next level. If you find an exercise too much of a challenge, you can substitute it with an alternative from a level below and the same movement pattern. Once you are competent with all of the featured exercises you can then include progressions to make the programme even harder, or add a little variety by selecting exercises from a range of levels.

Mobilization warm-up (»pp.44–55) 5–10 mins					
EXERCISE	LEVEL	PAGE	SETS	REPS	REST (SECS)
1. FLEXION EXERCISES (CHOOSE ONE...)					
Partner Ball Swap	5	108–09	2–3	10–12	30–60
Medicine Ball Slam	6	120	2–3	10–12	30–60
Exercise Ball Jack-knife	8	142	2–3	10–12	30–60
Hanging Toe Tuck	10	150	2–3	10–12	30–60
4. ISOMETRIC EXERCISES (CHOOSE ONE...)					
Kettlebell Round-body Swing	5	117	2–3	10–12	30–60
Exercise Ball Knee Tuck	7	130	2–3	10–12	30–60
Single-leg, Single-arm Cable Press	9	148–49	2–3	10–12	30–60
Plank Plate Push	10	152–53	2–3	10–12	30–60
7. ROTATION EXERCISES (CHOOSE ONE...)					
Standing Plate Twist	5	116	2–3	10–12	30–60
Medicine Ball Bridge	6	123	2–3	10–12	30–60
Suspended Single-arm Core Rotation	6	126	2–3	10–12	30–60
Pulley Lift	8	146–47	2–3	10–12	30–60

GN YOUR OWN" PROGRAMME (LEVELS 5-10)

EXERCISE	LEVEL	PAGE	SETS	REPS	REST (SECS)
2. EXTENSION EXERCISES (CHOOSE ONE...)					
Good Morning	5	112	2-3	10-12	30-60
Exercise Ball Back Extension	6	122	2-3	10-12	30-60
Medicine Ball Reverse Throw	6	121	2-3	10-12	30-60
GHD Back Extension	8	143	2-3	10-12	30-60
5. COMPLEX EXERCISES (CHOOSE ONE...)					
Suspended Pendulum	6	127	2-3	10-12	30-60
Suspended Oblique Crunch	7	135	2-3	10-12	30-60
Medicine Ball Chop	7	136	2-3	10-12	30-60
Turkish Get-up with Kettlebell	10	156-57	2-3	10-12	30-60
8. ISOMETRIC EXERCISES (CHOOSE ONE...)					
Mountain Climber	5	118	2-3	10-12	30-60
Kettlebell Swing	7	129	2-3	10-12	30-60
Core Board Rotation	7	131	2-3	10-12	30-60
Stepped Plank Walk	10	154-55	2-3	10-12	30-60

EXERCISE	LEVEL	PAGE	SETS	REPS	REST (SECS)
3. ROTATION EXERCISES (CHOOSE ONE...)					
O-bar Rotation	5	114-15	2-3	10-12	30-60
Russian Twist	6	119	2-3	10-12	30-60
Wall Side Throw	6	124-25	2-3	10-12	30-60
Pulley Chop	8	144-45	2-3	10-12	30-60
6. FLEXION EXERCISES (CHOOSE ONE...)					
Hanging Knee-up	5	110-11	2-3	10-12	30-60
Medicine Ball Slam	6	120	2-3	10-12	30-60
Pike	8	139	2-3	10-12	30-60
Stick Crunch	8	140-41	2-3	10-12	30-60

Foam roller exercises (»pp.44-45) and static stretching (»pp.166-71) 5-10 mins

DURATION
4-6 weeks

FREQUENCY
2-3 workouts per week; 1-2 days' rest between workouts

THE CORE CHALLENGE 300

The following programme can be used both as a simple test to assess the rate of progress of your training and as a fun addition to your existing regimen. Each programme requires you to perform a total of 300 repetitions in the quickest possible time, and will push both your core strength and your mental toughness to the very limit.

Whom is it suitable for?

The Core Challenge 300 is an excellent training tool for people of all abilities. With three stages of difficulty to increase the level of the challenge as you improve, you can use it as a test to monitor the progress of your training, or as a fun and motivational addition to your regimen. However, you should only attempt it if you are familiar with the exercises involved.

What are the benefits?

There are no set benefits as such. The programme is in essence a fun exercise and a great way to motivate and challenge your core and mental strength. You can compete against your previous results, or against friends, but you should set yourself goals and try to improve each time.

How will I progress?

While the ultimate aim is to complete all 300 repetitions of each stage without any rest, to give you an initial idea of your current ability level, you should begin by attempting the Foundation stage. If you find that you can complete it without rest, you should progress to the Intermediate level and repeat the assessment, and so on. If you cannot complete the test without rest, you can adjust it in two ways to help you progress in a structured way. The first option is to decide on a set period of rest (of up to 1 minute) between exercises. As you improve, you can reduce this rest by 5–10 seconds per session until you can complete the challenge without rest. The second option is to break the required repetitions into a programme of more manageable loads. For example, 50 sit-ups could become 5 x 10 sit-ups with 10 seconds rest between each of the 10 reps. You can then reduce this rest period by a second each session, until you can complete the challenge without rest.

FOUNDATION (LEVELS 1–3)					
Mobilization warm-up (>>pp.44–55) 5–10 mins					
EXERCISE	MOVEMENT	PAGE	SETS	REPS	REST (SECS)
Sit-up	F	78	1	50	–
Dorsal Raise	E	76–77	1	25	–
Oblique Reach	R	86–87	1	25	–
Reverse Curl	F	75	1	25	–
Abdominal Crunch	F	72–73	1	50	–
Super-slow Bicycle	R	95	1	25	–
Sprinter Sit-up	F	96	1	25	–
Superman	F	70–71	1	25	–
Sit-up	F	78	1	50	–
Foam roller exercises (>>pp.44–45) and static stretching (>>pp.166–71) 5–10 mins					

DURATION OF PROGRAMME
4–6 weeks

FREQUENCY OF PROGRAMME
As required, but with 1–2 days' rest between workouts

INTERMEDIATE (LEVELS 4–6)

Mobilization warm-up (>>pp.44–55) 5–10 mins

EXERCISE	MOVEMENT	PAGE	SETS	REPS	REST (SECS)
Kettlebell Round-body Swing	I	117	1	50	–
Medicine Ball Slam	F	120	1	25	–
O-bar Rotation	R	114–15	1	25	–
Hanging Knee-up	F	110–11	1	25	–
Kettlebell Swing	I	129	1	50	–
Mountain Climber	I	118	1	25	–
Russian Twist	R	119	1	25	–
Exercise Ball Knee Tuck	I	130	1	25	–
Medicine Ball Chop	C	136	1	50	–

Foam roller exercises (>>pp.44–45)
and static stretching (>>pp.166–71) 5–10 mins

DURATION OF PROGRAMME
4–6 weeks

FREQUENCY OF PROGRAMME
As required, but with 1–2 days' rest between workouts

ADVANCED (LEVELS 7–10)

Mobilization warm-up (>>pp.44–55) 5–10 mins

EXERCISE	MOVEMENT	PAGE	SETS	REPS	REST (SECS)
Sandbag Shouldering	C	151	1	50	–
Stick Crunch	F	140–41	1	25	–
Exercise Ball Hip Rotation Kick	C	158–59	1	25	–
Hanging Toe Tuck	F	150	1	25	–
Pulley Chop	R	144–45	1	50	–
Exercise Ball Jack-knife	F	142	1	25	–
Raised Pike Dumbbell Hand-walk	C	162–63	1	25	–
Plank Plate Push	F	152–53	1	25	–
Turkish Get-up with Kettlebell	C	156–57	1	50	–

Foam roller exercises (>>pp.44–45)
and static stretching (>>pp.166–71) 5–10 mins

DURATION OF PROGRAMME
4–6 weeks

FREQUENCY OF PROGRAMME
As required, but with 1–2 days' rest between workouts

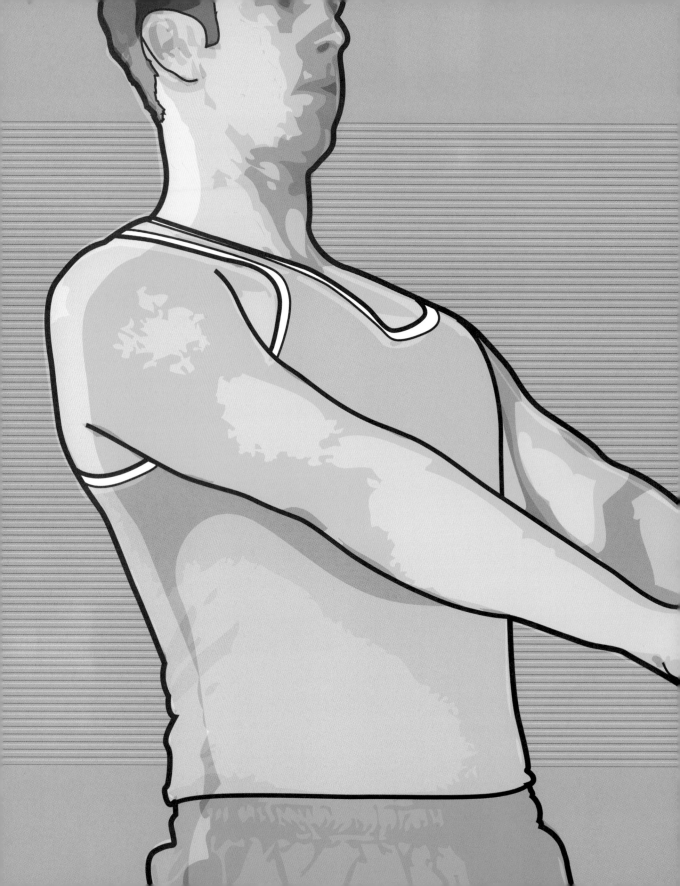

SPORTS-SPECIFIC CORE TRAINING

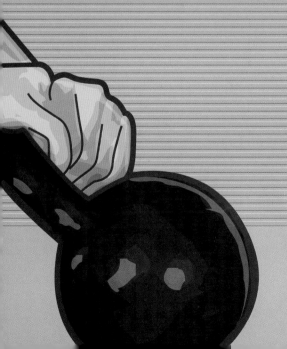

4

INTRODUCTION

The term "sports-specific" is applied to any form of training that is specifically tailored to the needs of an individual sport. In practice, this means that the training requirements of an individual athlete are first analyzed according to the specific movement patterns of their particular sport. These movement patterns are then replicated in the athlete's training regimen with the aim of optimizing their performance.

THE IMPORTANCE OF THE CORE TO SPORT

Good core strength plays an essential role in achieving optimal performance in your chosen sport. Since the core is the foundation of all bodily movements, training it to work effectively helps you to achieve the kinds of fast and powerful body movements required by your sport, and reduces your risk of injury because it helps your muscles and joints to function more efficiently.

The muscles of your core are involved in the most basic of day-to-day movements – from bending down to pick something off the ground to climbing the stairs. For the sportsperson, however, the core is vital, no matter what movements are involved. In golf, for example, the swing of a club involves the transfer of stress from the back and shoulders to the core in order to control and perfect the movement, while reducing the risk of straining. In kayaking, likewise, the core directs and maintains the transfer of power to the shoulders and arms, driving the paddling stroke as efficiently as possible. And in gymnastics, core strength is essential for achieving and holding the numerous body positions required.

THE PLANES OF MOVEMENT

Whatever your chosen sport, you should always ensure that you train your core in all planes of movement (»p.26) in order to achieve the maximum possible level of strength, stability, and mobility. Most sports involve a combination of complex movements, involving all three planes of movement, and so training in this way will dramatically increase your sporting performance, with obvious positive benefits to your balance, co-ordination, strength, stamina, and general level of technique.

USING THE SPORTS-SPECIFIC MATRIX

The sports-specific matrix charts featured over the next three pages provide a breakdown of individual sports according to the characteristic movement patterns involved in each. The movement patterns are categorized in terms of their relevance as follows: primary movement (**black square**); secondary or general movement (**clear square**); and no relevance (**blank**). Isometric strength, for example, is important in a wide range of sports, but especially those that involve grappling with an opponent or resisting an external force, such as in rugby or weightlifting. Flexion and extension strength, meanwhile, are key to sports like basketball or volleyball, which involve bending, and reaching or jumping. Rotation and side flexion are especially important in sports that require good rotational power, such as tennis or martial arts. And, while complex core movements are relevant to most sports, they are particularly important in sports that involve explosive, multi-directional movements, such as football and ice hockey. The information in this table can be used in conjunction with the Exercises by Movement Matrix (»pp.40–43), which provides a list of exercises grouped by movement type and difficulty level.

THE SPORTS-SPECIFIC MATRIX

The sports-specific matrix in this section (»pp.195–97) features some of the more dominant movement patterns you may want to consider when devising training programmes for your sport. However, if a particular core movement is not featured in the matrix, it does not mean that it is not necessary. As highlighted earlier, all sports require a good overall level of core strength, and this only comes from training all of the core's movement patterns. And so, you should aim for a "complete" core training programme to reduce the likelihood of muscular imbalance and the risk of injury, while also focusing on the movement patterns applicable to your sport.

WARNING!

Before you begin any form of sports-specific core training, you must have a solid foundation of core strength, stability, and mobility. This means you should be able to complete all of the exercises in the Foundation, Activation, and Intermediate sections (»pp.56–137) and the Fundamental Core Strength programme (»pp.176–177) with good technique. You should also always seek the advice of a qualified coach (»pp.224) before you begin.

SPORTS-SPECIFIC MATRIX

Key
The six core movements (>>p.9; p.27) are listed on the right. Below are the sports they are relevant to. The key is:
- ■ Direct relevance
- □ Partial / general relevance

	Isometric	Flexion	Extension	Side flexion	Rotation	Complex
American / Canadian football	■	□	□	□	■	□
Australian rules football	■	□	□	□	■	□
Badminton	□	■	□	■	■	□
Baseball / softball	□	□	□	■	■	□
Basketball	■	□	□	□	■	□
BMX biking	■	□	□	■	■	□
Boxing	□	■	□	■	■	□
Canoeing	■			□	■	
Climbing	■	□	□	□	□	■
Cricket	□	□	□	□	■	
Cross-country running	■	■	■	□	■	
Cycling	■		■	■	■	■
Dinghy sailing	■				■	
Discus	■	□	□	□	■	□
Distance running	■	■	■	□	■	
Diving	■	■	■	■	■	■
Dodgeball	□	□	□	□	■	■
Dressage	■				□	
Eventing	■				□	
Fencing	■	□	□	□		
Field hockey	□				■	
Gaelic football	□	□	□		■	■
Golf	□			□	■	
Gymnastics	■	■	■	■	■	■
Hammer	■	□	□	□	■	□
Handball	■	□	□		■	□
High jump	□	■	■		□	■
Horse riding	■			□		

Key
The six core movements (>>p.9; p.27) are listed on the right. Below are the sports they are relevant to. The key is:
■ Direct relevance
□ Partial / general relevance

	Isometric	Flexion	Extension	Side flexion	Rotation	Complex
Hurling	□	□	□		■	■
Ice climbing	■	□	□	■	□	■
Ice hockey	■	□	□	□	■	■
Ice skating	■	□	□	□	□	
Javelin	■	□	□	□	■	■
Judo	■	■	■	■	■	■
Ju-jitsu	■	■	■	■	■	■
Karate	■	■	■	■	■	■
Kayaking	■				■	
Kickboxing	■	■	■	■	■	■
Kitesurfing	■	■	■	■	■	■
Korfball	□	□	□		□	■
Kung fu	■	■	■	■	■	■
Lacrosse	■	□	□		■	□
Long-distance running	■	■	■	□	□	
Long jump / triple jump	■	□	□	□	■	
Middle-distance running	■	■	■	□	■	
Mixed martial arts	■	■	■	■	■	
Mountaineering	■	□	□			■
Mountain biking	■			□	□	
Netball	□	□	□		□	■
Parkour	■	■	■	■	■	■
Pole vault	■	■	■		■	■
Polo	■			□	■	
Powerlifting	■	■	■	■		■
Real tennis	■	□	□	□	■	□
Road racing (bicycle)	■			■	■	
Rock climbing	■	□	□	□	□	■
Rollerblading	■			□	■	
Rollerskating	■			□	■	

Key

The six core movements (>>p.9; p.27) are listed on the right. Below are the sports they are relevant to. The key is:

■ Direct relevance
☐ Partial / general relevance

	Isometric	Flexion	Extension	Side flexion	Rotation	Complex
Rounders	☐	☐	☐		■	
Rowing	■	☐	☐		☐	
Rugby league	■	■	■	☐	■	■
Rugby union	■	■	■	☐	■	■
Sculling	■	☐	☐		☐	
Shot put	■	☐	☐	☐	■	☐
Showjumping	■			☐		
Skateboarding	■			☐		
Skiing	■			☐	■	
Skydiving	■					
Snowboarding	■			☐	■	
Soccer	☐	■	■		☐	
Speed-skating	■	☐	☐	☐	■	■
Sprints	■	■	■	☐	☐	
Squash / racketball	■			☐	■	☐
Steeplechase (horse)	■	■	■	☐	☐	
Striking martial arts	■	■	■	■	■	■
Surfing	■			☐		
Swimming	■	☐	☐		■	☐
Taekwondo	■	■	■	■	■	■
Table tennis	■	☐	☐	☐	■	☐
Tennis	☐	■	☐	■	■	☐
Track cycling	■			☐	■	
Volleyball	■	☐	☐		■	☐
Waterskiing	■			☐	☐	
Water polo	■	☐	☐		■	☐
Whitewater rafting	■	☐	☐	☐	■	
Weightlifting	■	■	■	■		■
Windsurfing	■	☐	☐	☐	☐	
Wrestling	■	☐	☐	☐	■	■

COLLISION TEAM SPORTS

Collision team sports involve a combination of explosive multi-directional movements and high-impact contact with opponents. Players therefore require excellent strength, stability, and mobility.

All powerful movements are generated in your core. Building good core stability is therefore important because it provides a solid and stable platform from which to transfer this power to your limbs, maximizing the efficiency of movements such as throwing, kicking, and tackling. Combined with core mobility, it ensures a strong, stable, and mobile foundation for actions such as goalkeeping, catching, and resisting tackles, while improving your agility and balance, and reducing your risk of injury.

Good rotational strength improves throwing

A strong core provides a powerbase for your limbs, and helps you to fend off opponents

SPORTS SUCH AS...

- American football
- Aussie rules football
- Rugby league
- Rugby union
- Ice hockey
- Gaelic football
- Lacrosse
- Hurling

CORE-STRENGTH TRAINING FOR COLLISION TEAM SPORTS

All collision team sports utilize complex movements, so you should train your core according to the demands of the sport and the dominant core movements involved. Training should focus on total fitness, preparing for games with a combination of strength-training circuits to develop power and interval training to improve cardiovascular fitness.

PREPARATION
Warm-ups, both for training and for matches, should include dynamic stretches and cardiovascular work, such as shuttle runs, to raise the temperature of your body. Cool-downs should include gentle jogging and stretching to reduce muscle tightness.

■ **Isometric**
Isometric exercises like planks (»pp.102–05) help to build your isometric strength and core stability, establishing a strong foundation for generating power and helping you resist the force of opponents.

■ **Rotation**
Rotational exercises such as wall side throws (»pp.124–25) improve your rotational power, helping with the speed and power of your kicks and passes, and stabilizing your body against torsional movements in contact.

■ **Flexion**
Flexion exercises such as medicine ball slams (»p.120) help you to develop power and mobility in your hips, improving your kicking ability and the downward force needed to grapple with opponents.

CONTACT SPORTS

Contact team sports require high levels of speed and agility combined with strength to fend off opponents in contact situations and the ability to deliver controlled power from unbalanced body positions.

Good core stability and mobility play an important role in helping you cope with the demands of twisting, turning, and changing direction – often at high speed – that are common in contact sports. Core stability and strength provide a stable platform from which to bring a ball under control, and help generate controlled power in passes and shots from unstable body positions and when under pressure from opponents. Core strength also helps you to resist the impact of contact with opponents and limits the risk of injury.

Core stability improves your overall balance

Core flexion can help with speed and kicking power

SPORTS SUCH AS...

- Football
- Handball
- Dodgeball
- Field hockey

CORE-STRENGTH TRAINING FOR CONTACT SPORTS

All contact sports require excellent cardiovascular fitness and a range of complex movements. Training should involve a combination of interval training to improve cardiovascular fitness and strength-training circuits to develop muscular power. The latter should focus on the muscles specific to your sport.

PREPARATION
Good warm-up and cool-down procedures on match days, and a training programme that offers preparation for games, are essential. Warm-ups should include dynamic stretches and cardiovascular work, such as shuttle runs, to raise your body temperature.

■ Isometric
Isometric exercises such as mountain climbers (»p.118) help build your core stability. This provides a solid platform for coping with multi-directional movements, controlling shots and passes, and fending off opponents.

■ Rotation
Rotational exercises such as pulley lifts (»pp.146–47) improve your rotational power. This increases the power of your kicks and passes, and stabilizes your body against torsional movements in contact.

■ Flexion
Flexion exercises such as partner ball swaps (»pp.108–09) help you to generate greater hip strength and mobility, improving your control and power when you are passing or shooting.

NET-BASED SPORTS

The frequent jumping and landing involved in net-based sports require high levels of stamina and cardiovascular fitness. Core stability is also crucial in holding the body in a stationary position when taking shots.

Although contact is limited in net-based sports, twisting, turning, and pivoting movements are common, either to make a pass or to shake off an opponent. These carry the risk of strain-related injury to vulnerable joints, such as your ankles and knees. Developing your core stability and mobility will help to improve your balance, making over-extension injuries less likely. Training to increase strength in your core will also help you to generate the explosive power required to make short sprints up and down the court, or to drive past an opponent.

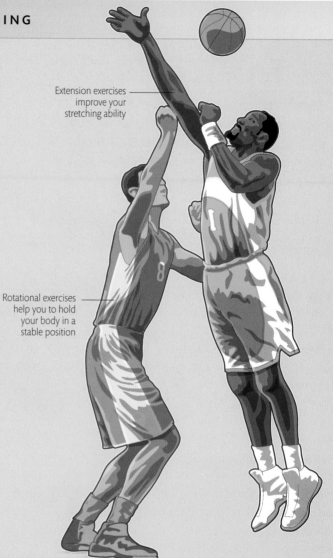

Extension exercises improve your stretching ability

Rotational exercises help you to hold your body in a stable position

SPORTS SUCH AS...

- Basketball
- Netball
- Korfball
- Volleyball

CORE-STRENGTH TRAINING FOR NET-BASED SPORTS

A core-training programme for net-based sports should combine flexion and extension exercises to improve flexibility and balance, with exercises to build rotational strength. Interval training will improve your cardiovascular fitness, preparing you for the sprints required to cover the court.

PREPARATION
Warm-ups should include dynamic stretches as well as cardiovascular work, such as shuttle runs, to raise your body temperature. Cool-downs should include gentle jogging and stretching to stop your muscles from seizing up.

■ Flexion
Flexion exercises such as partner ball swaps (**»pp.108–09**) help you to generate greater hip strength and mobility, improving your power and control, along with your ability to reach the ball, especially when it is close to the ground.

■ Extension
Extension exercises such as medicine ball reverse throws (**»p.121**) improve your spinal mobility and stability. This helps you to stretch when catching and to hold your torso in a stationary position when shooting or passing.

■ Rotation
Rotational exercises such as standing plate twists (**»p.116**) improve your rotational strength and mobility. This increases the power and distance of your throws, and further helps to stabilize your body.

BAT- AND CLUB-BASED SPORTS

Bat- and club-based sports demand focused rotational power and control. Good core stability plays an important role as it helps players to hold their bodies in the optimum position for taking shots.

Although developing power in your core will enable you to hit the ball further, core training can also help to improve your shot-making technique. If some of your muscles are over-developed, there is a chance that they will take over the work of weaker muscles in an effort to generate more power, resulting in distortions in your stroke. Because poor technique is responsible for the majority of mis-hits and back injuries, a well-rounded core-training program that reduces the likelihood of muscle imbalances is likely to result in improved performance and a reduced risk of injury.

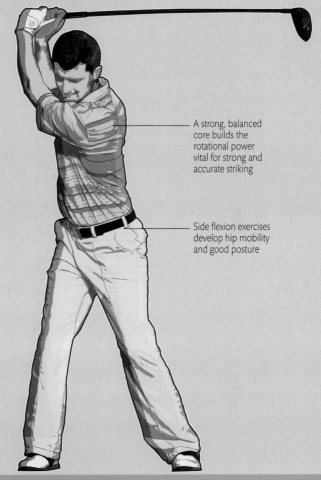

A strong, balanced core builds the rotational power vital for strong and accurate striking

Side flexion exercises develop hip mobility and good posture

SPORTS SUCH AS...

- Baseball
- Softball
- Rounders
- Cricket
- Golf

CORE-STRENGTH TRAINING FOR BAT- AND CLUB-BASED SPORTS

Much of the training in bat- and club-based sports focuses on technique, but strength and fitness should come first. Combine cardiovascular work with strength-training circuits to develop general fitness and to increase your power. Do also practise sprinting; most bat- and club-based sports involve short sprints interspersed with long recovery times.

PREPARATION
Warm-ups should involve dynamic stretches that imitate the movements required by your particular sport. Cool-downs should include a range of static stretches to reduce muscle tightness and reduce the risk of them seizing up.

■ Rotation
Rotational exercises such as pulley chops (**»pp.144–45**) build your rotational strength and mobility. This helps to improve the quality of your stroke, and increase the power, range, and accuracy of your shots.

■ Isometric
Isometric exercises such as kettlebell round-body swings (**»p.117**) help you to generate greater stability and strength in your core and pelvis. This enables you to hold your body in the correct position when striking or pitching the ball.

■ Side flexion
Side flexion exercises such as windmills (**»pp.110–11**) improve your spinal mobility and stability, further aiding your ability to hold your body in the optimum striking position.

RACKET-BASED SPORTS

Racket-based sports demand great agility and cardiovascular fitness, requiring players to return shots with high speed and accuracy, often when off-balance.

The majority of shots in racket-based sports are played with the arm positioned to the side of the body. The arm muscles cannot generate much power on their own, so the best way to put force behind your shots is by using your core rotational strength. Improving your flexion will allow you to reach further for the ball from a stable base, while retaining power and accuracy in your shots.

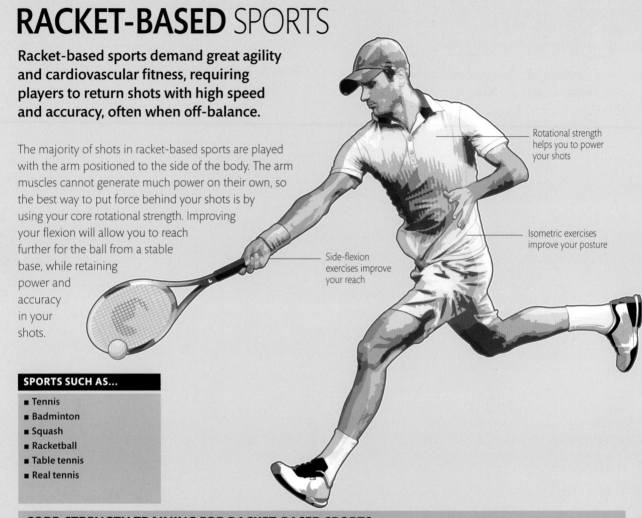

Rotational strength helps you to power your shots

Isometric exercises improve your posture

Side-flexion exercises improve your reach

SPORTS SUCH AS...

- Tennis
- Badminton
- Squash
- Racketball
- Table tennis
- Real tennis

CORE-STRENGTH TRAINING FOR RACKET-BASED SPORTS

A core-training programme for racket-based sports should combine exercises to build your rotational strength with isometric and side flexion exercises to improve your flexibility and balance. Interval training will improve your cardiovascular fitness, preparing you for the sprints required to cover the court.

PREPARATION
Warm-ups should involve dynamic stretches that imitate the movements required by your particular sport. Cool-downs should combine gentle jogging with static stretches to stop your muscles getting tight or seizing up.

■ Rotation
Rotational exercises such as pulley chops (**»pp.144–45**) improve your rotational strength and mobility, and help to stabilize your spine. They are especially beneficial when it comes to achieving an optimum serve.

■ Side flexion
Side-flexion exercises such as side bends (**»p.81**) improve your spinal mobility and stability. These generate power and control in your limbs as well as help with the movements involved in stretching to reach awkward shots.

■ Isometric
Isometric exercises such as single-leg, single-arm cable presses (**»pp.148–49**) build core stability and strength. These enable you to hold your body in the correct position and improve the accuracy of your shots.

RUNNING

While cardiovascular fitness is a priority for runners, good posture is also vital. This reduces lateral movement and improves the speed and efficiency of the runner's stride, reducing the risk of injury.

Core stability reduces unwanted secondary movement, such as the unintended side-to-side sway of a runner's torso. These small movements are a major obstacle to achieving maximum performance – both for short- and long-distance runners – since they reduce momentum by diverting energy from its intended purpose, placing uncontrolled strain on the body and potentially causing injury. For athletes who run on uneven surfaces (cross-country or road runners, for example) core training improves posture and spinal alignment with positive benefits for balance.

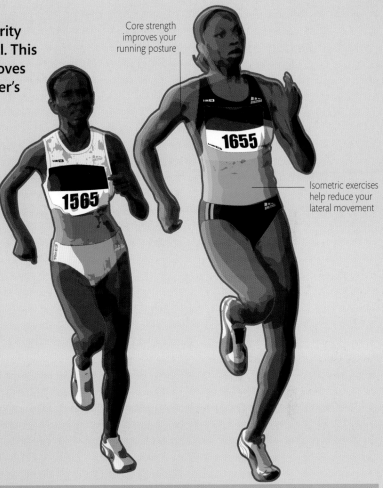

Core strength improves your running posture

Isometric exercises help reduce your lateral movement

SPORTS SUCH AS...

- Sprinting
- Middle-distance running
- Long-distance running
- Cross-country running

CORE-STRENGTH TRAINING FOR RUNNING

Running can be hard on your knees and ankles, so in addition to your regular running programme, a low-impact exercise such as swimming is a good way of maintaining all-round fitness while giving your joints time to recover. A stretching routine is also essential before and after running to reduce stiffness and help prevent injury.

PREPARATION
Warm-ups for running should involve dynamic stretches to prepare your body for strenuous activity. Cool-downs should include static stretches to lengthen your muscles and prevent them from seizing up.

 ■ **Isometric**
Isometric exercises such as mountain climbers (》p.118) build core stability and strength. This enables you to achieve an optimal body position when running, taking the strain off your back and hips.

 ■ **Extension**
Extension exercises such as GHD back extensions (》p.143) improve back and hip alignment and mobility, and strengthen hip placement, minimizing the stress placed on your joints as a result of running.

 ■ **Rotation**
Rotational exercises such as o-bar rotations (》pp.114–15) improve your rotational strength and mobility. This increases the speed at which you can roll your hips, and so increases running speed.

THROWING-BASED FIELD SPORTS

Throwing-based field sports demand a combination of speed, explosive rotational power, and control, all of which depend on good core stability.

Core strength provides a platform from which to generate the power needed for throwing, and to deliver it efficiently without unnecessary lateral movement. It also enables athletes to better achieve the best possible body position, and to turn around from the waist even from an unstable standing position. Javelin throwers need speed in their hip flexors for their run-up, and are advised to train using flexion exercises, while discus throwers benefit from rotational exercises. Hammer throwers and shot putters use both rotational and isometric exercises as these give them the core strength they need to hold a fixed position while briefly resisting the force of the particular weight they are about to throw.

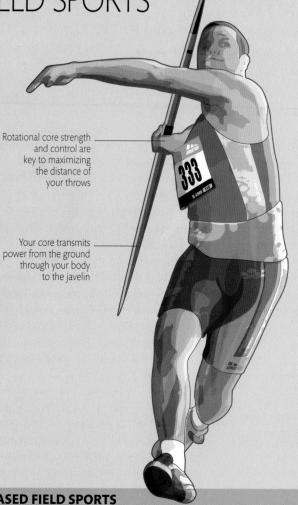

Rotational core strength and control are key to maximizing the distance of your throws

Your core transmits power from the ground through your body to the javelin

SPORTS SUCH AS...

- Baseball
- Discus
- Cricket
- Hammer
- Javelin
- Shot put

CORE-STRENGTH TRAINING FOR THROWING-BASED FIELD SPORTS

A core-training programme for throwing-based field sports should combine flexion and extension exercises, to improve your flexibility and balance, with exercises to build your rotational strength. Combine upper-body workouts with core-stability exercises to maximize both the generation and the efficient transfer of rotational power.

PREPARATION
Warm-ups should involve dynamic stretches that imitate the movement required by the throwing sport you are practising. Cool-downs should take the form of static stretches and some light jogging to prevent your muscles from seizing up.

■ Rotation
Exercises such as Russian twists (»p.119) help improve rotational strength and mobility, increasing the power and distance of throws, and helping stabilize your torso to maximize the transfer of power from your core to your throwing arm.

■ Flexion
Flexion exercises like medicine ball slams (»p.120) help you to generate greater core strength and mobility, improving your explosive power and control, and easing the shift of energy from your core to your throwing arm.

■ Isometric
Isometric exercises such as ball knee tucks (»p.130) help build stability and strength in your core and pelvis and maintain body position when throwing, improving control and power and reducing the risk of injury.

JUMPING-BASED FIELD SPORTS

Jumping-based field sports demand a mixture of explosive power, mobility, and core control in order to jump as far, or as high, as possible.

Flexion exercises help athletes achieve explosive power in their take-offs, while extension movements help in stretching the body to gain precious extra centimetres, or in bending back to lift over a high-jump bar. The latter exercises also help make over-extension injuries less likely. In carrying out the triple jump, developing rotational power is important, while training to increase strength in your core will also help you to generate the energy required in run-ups. Good plyometric and acceleration fitness is also crucial for this, as it helps ensure you can achieve the perfect speed when you take off.

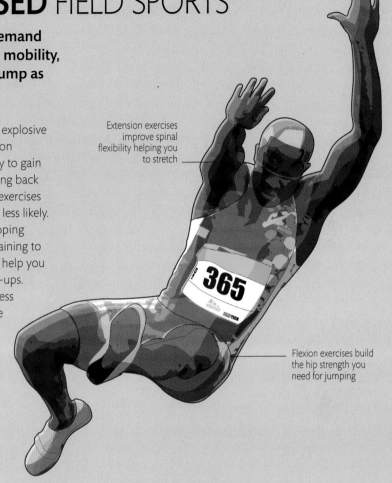

Extension exercises improve spinal flexibility helping you to stretch

Flexion exercises build the hip strength you need for jumping

SPORTS SUCH AS...

- High jump
- Long jump
- Pole vault
- Triple jump

CORE-STRENGTH TRAINING FOR JUMPING-BASED FIELD SPORTS

Your core-training programme for jumping-based sports should combine flexion and extension exercises to improve flexibility and balance with exercises to build isometric and rotational strength. Interval training will improve your cardiovascular fitness, preparing you for the sprints that are required in run-ups.

PREPARATION

Warm-ups for jumping activities should involve dynamic stretches to prepare your body for bursts of strenuous activity. Cool-downs should include light jogging and static stretching to prevent your muscles from getting tight.

■ Flexion
Flexion exercises such as hanging toe tucks (**»p.150**) will help you generate greater hip strength and improve mobility and strength of the core. This will improve explosive power, mobility, and control in both your hips and spine.

■ Extension
Extension exercises such as medicine ball reverse throws (**»p.121**) improve your spinal mobility, stability, and strength, which will help you to stretch and curve your spine, which is especially important in the high jump and pole vault.

■ Rotation
Rotational exercises such as standing plate twists (**»p.116**) help to improve your rotational strength, mobility, and spinal control, which are vital for the turning movements involved in the high jump.

WEIGHTLIFTING AND POWERLIFTING

Weightlifting and powerlifting put huge amounts of stress on the joints and work muscles to their limit. Excellent core stability is crucial to generate the power, speed, and control needed for a successful lift.

Flexion and extension exercises should be the focus of any good core-strength training programme for weightlifters. Improving the flexion of your lumbar spine will make bending to pick up the weight easier, while performing extension exercises will improve your final locking-out movement. Isometric exercises will increase your ability to brace your body against the weight of a load and hold the weight in a static position once you have lifted it above your head.

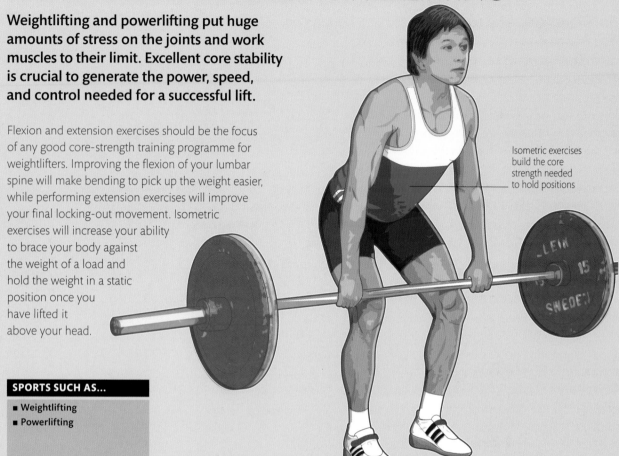

Isometric exercises build the core strength needed to hold positions

SPORTS SUCH AS...

- Weightlifting
- Powerlifting

CORE-STRENGTH TRAINING FOR WEIGHTLIFTING AND POWERLIFTING

Intersperse your strength training with light cardiovascular exercise, such as gentle jogging or swimming, which will help to stretch and lengthen your muscles.

Dynamic stretches, in which you complete a full range of motion without stopping, will mobilize your muscles, minimizing stiffness and reducing the risk of injury.

PREPARATION
Warm-ups for weightlifting and powerlifting should involve dynamic stretches that imitate the movements required and prepare your body for strenuous activity. Cool-downs should feature static stretches to prevent muscles from seizing up.

■ Extension
Using extension exercises like good mornings (»pp.112–13) improve your spinal stability and strength, helping you to hold a lift with good form when you raise the weight above your head.

■ Flexion
Flexion exercises such as the double-leg extension and stretch (»p.107) help you to generate greater hip strength and mobility, improving your power and stability in the crouching and standing phases of a lift.

■ Isometric
Isometric exercises such as core board rotations (»p.131) build your core stability and strength. These enable you to hold your body in the correct position during the acceleration and standing phases of the lift.

COMBAT SPORTS

Combat sports require a combination of speed, strength, stamina, explosive power, and agility, all of which can be improved through a core-training programme.

Building your core rotational strength will increase the power of your punches, kicks, and throws, as well as enhancing your ability to withstand blows to your body. Working on side flexion will make it easier for you to evade blows by ducking and weaving, and will improve your pelvic and spinal alignment. Good alignment will make it harder for you to be caught off-balance.

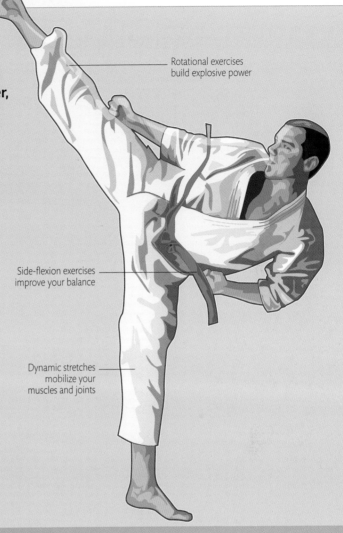

Rotational exercises build explosive power

Side-flexion exercises improve your balance

Dynamic stretches mobilize your muscles and joints

SPORTS SUCH AS...

- Boxing
- Fencing
- Karate
- Kung fu
- Judo
- Ju-jitsu
- Kickboxing
- Mixed martial arts
- Wrestling
- Taekwondo

CORE-STRENGTH TRAINING FOR COMBAT SPORTS

Meeting the range of demands made by combat sports requires a varied training programme that builds strength and develops cardiovascular fitness. Draw up a programme of strength-training circuits to increase your explosive power and endurance, and plan a course of dynamic stretches to lengthen and loosen the muscles.

PREPARATION

Warm-ups for combat sports should involve dynamic stretches that imitate the movements required and prepare your body for strenuous activity. Cool-downs should include static stretches to prevent tight muscles.

■ Isometric
Isometric exercises such as side planks (**»pp.104–05**) build core stability, enabling you to hold your body in a fixed position despite external force. This is useful for resisting being knocked off balance, for example.

■ Rotation
Rotational exercises such as medicine ball bridges (**»p.123**) improve your rotational mobility. This increases both the power of your punches and your ability to throw an opponent, and helps you to resist your opponent's blows.

■ Side flexion
Side flexion exercises such as windmills (**»pp.110–11**) improve your spinal mobility and stability. This benefits your balance and increases your skill at ducking and weaving to evade your opponents.

BOARD-BASED SPORTS

Board-based sports require great strength of the legs, hips, and ankles, as well as core strength for bracing against a constantly changing terrain.

Exercises to build isometric strength will help to brace your body against the external forces exerted on the body by waves or uneven terrain. Practising side-flexion exercises will improve the stability of your stance when your torso and legs are not aligned. Developing your rotational core strength will have a beneficial effect on your ability to control the board by transferring force from the hips through your legs and into your feet.

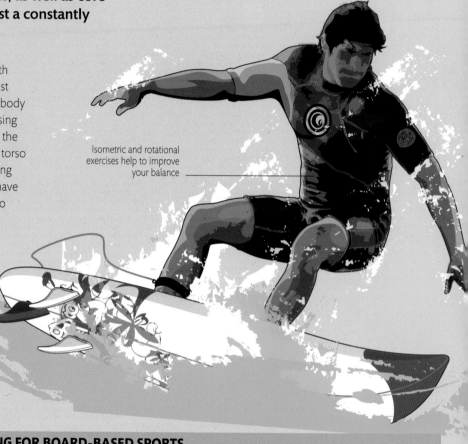

Isometric and rotational exercises help to improve your balance

SPORTS SUCH AS...

- **Surfing**
- **Windsurfing**
- **Snowboarding**
- **Skateboarding**
- **Kitesurfing**

CORE-STRENGTH TRAINING FOR BOARD-BASED SPORTS

Your legs are key to control in board-based sports. Consequently, weight-training circuits with an emphasis on developing strength in your legs will have a beneficial effect on your performance. As well as maintaining cardiovascular fitness, a cycling programme will help to build strength in leg muscles such as the quadriceps and the calves.

PREPARATION
Warm-ups should involve dynamic stretches that imitate the movements required by your particular sport. Cool-downs should include a range of static stretches to help stop your muscles getting tight or seizing up.

■ Isometric
Isometric exercises such as supermans (**»pp.70–71**) build core stability, strength, and balance, helping you to improve your movement over difficult and constantly varying terrain.

■ Rotation
Exercises such as O-bar rotations (**»pp.114–15**) improve rotational strength, stability, and mobility, working in combination with your isometric strength to give you excellent balance and control of your core.

■ Side flexion
Side-flexion exercises such as Roman chair side-bends (**»p.83**) improve your spinal mobility and stability, further aiding your ability to hold your body in a balanced position.

GYMNASTICS

Gymnastics requires cardiovascular fitness, core strength, and suppleness throughout the body. More than any other sport, it involves technical manoeuvres that should only be learned one step at a time.

Running, swimming, and interval training are all good cardiovascular exercises that will help you to build the stamina needed to practise your particular discipline. Otherwise, training should focus on attaining a high level of flexibility as well as complex, multi-directional joint mobility. Spinal stability is vital, and for this a combination of flexion, isometric, and extension exercises is recommended. Isometric strength is particularly important for holding difficult positions on the floor, rings, or pommel horse.

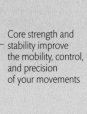

Core strength and stability improve the mobility, control, and precision of your movements

POMMEL HSE
POMMEL HSE   POMMEL HSE

SPORTS SUCH AS...

- **Acrobatic gymnastics**
- **Aerobic gymnastics**
- **Artistic gymnastics**
- **Display gymnastics**
- **Rhythmic gymnastics**
- **Trampolining and tumbling**

CORE-STRENGTH TRAINING FOR GYMNASTICS

Training your body for gymnastics should involve a programme of exercises that promote explosive power in the muscles. Improving all-round cardiovascular fitness through interval training will also help, as will exercises that strengthen your back. Flexibility can develop through extensive stretching, yoga, and Pilates programmes.

PREPARATION
Warm-ups should involve cardiovascular work to raise your body temperature and dynamic stretches that imitate the movements in your particular discipline. Cool-downs should involve light jogging and static stretches to prevent tight muscles.

■ Isometric
Exercises such as stepped plank walks (**»pp.154–55**) help to build core strength and engage the muscles of your lower and upper body. This will train your body to stabilize and support your limb weight and movement.

■ Extension
Extension exercises such as good mornings (**»pp.112–13**) help to stabilize and strengthen your spine and generate better power and control by improving your hip and leg strength and mobility.

■ Flexion
Flexion exercises such as hanging toe tucks (**»p.150**) help to build strength and power in your abdominals and hips, especially when lifting and supporting lower-body weight, which is vital for all types of gymnastics.

SKI- AND SKATE-BASED SPORTS

A strong core and cardiovascular fitness are essential for success in ski- and skate-based sports, which work muscles throughout the body. Balance and posture are particularly important, especially when travelling over difficult terrain.

SPORTS SUCH AS...

- Skiing
- Waterskiing
- Ice skating
- Speed skating
- Roller skating
- Roller blading
- Ice hockey

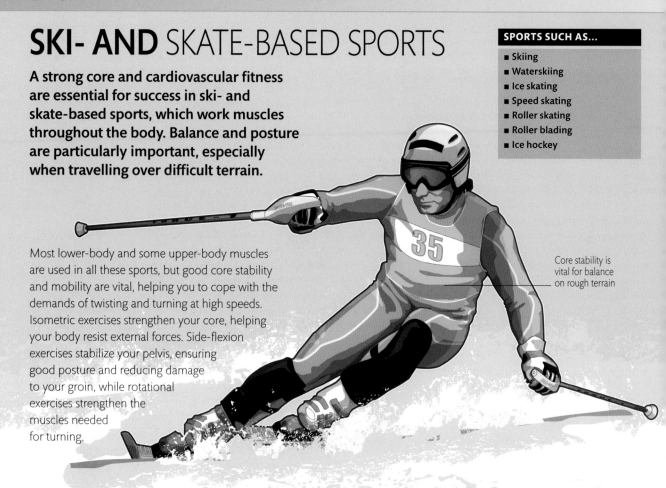

Most lower-body and some upper-body muscles are used in all these sports, but good core stability and mobility are vital, helping you to cope with the demands of twisting and turning at high speeds. Isometric exercises strengthen your core, helping your body resist external forces. Side-flexion exercises stabilize your pelvis, ensuring good posture and reducing damage to your groin, while rotational exercises strengthen the muscles needed for turning.

Core stability is vital for balance on rough terrain

CORE-STRENGTH TRAINING FOR SKI- AND SKATE-BASED SPORTS

Interval training is a good way of developing cardiovascular fitness, while mobility exercises are important for avoiding sprains and strains. Exercises that emphasize core strength will allow your pelvis to transfer power to your lower limbs without overly straining your body, thus reducing the risk of injury.

PREPARATION
Warm-ups should involve gentle cardiovascular exercises to prevent muscle strain caused by rapid changes of pace. Cool-downs should include jogging and static stretches to stretch your muscles.

■ Isometric
Isometric exercises such as kettlebell round-body swings (»p.117) help build core stability and strength, allowing you to balance when travelling over difficult and varying terrain. They also help to stabilize your spine.

■ Rotation
Rotational exercises such as pulley chops (»pp.144–45) improve your rotational strength, stability, and mobility. These give you excellent balance and control, which are vital for moving in ever-changing directions.

■ Side flexion
Exercises such as heel reaches (»p.82) help your spinal mobility and stability, further aiding your ability to hold your body in a balanced position, and enabling you to turn and lean while moving fast.

WATER SPORTS

Good technique, fostered by a core-training programme, is key to success in water sports such as kayaking and canoeing, which put great strain on the back, shoulders, forearms, and wrists.

SPORTS SUCH AS...
- Kayaking
- Canoeing
- Dinghy sailing
- Whitewater rafting
- Rowing
- Sculling

Isometric and rotational strength training condition your body to resist the force of moving water. Maintaining the correct posture, with your body stable and balanced, keeps you upright and makes it easier for you to transmit power from your arms and legs when paddling or rowing. For canoers, kayakers, and rafters, side-flexion strength combined with good core stability are vital for remaining upright even when the force of the water rolls you to the side.

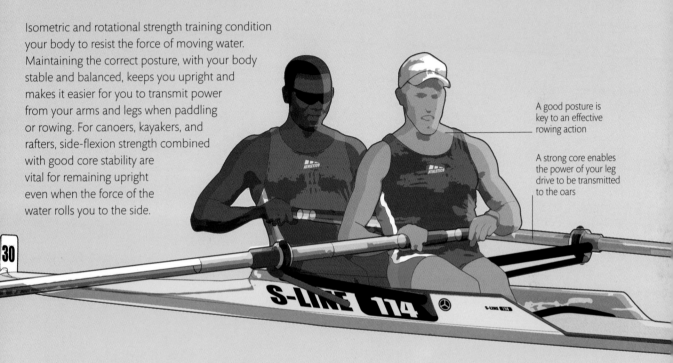

A good posture is key to an effective rowing action

A strong core enables the power of your leg drive to be transmitted to the oars

CORE-STRENGTH TRAINING FOR WATER SPORTS

Being able to sustain high levels of effort for a prolonged period of time is key to many water sports. A cardiovascular programme involving interval training will help you to achieve greater levels of endurance. In addition, strength-training circuits will increase the power in your torso and arms.

PREPARATION
Warm-ups should involve cardiovascular work such as gentle jogging and some stretches that imitate the movements used in your particular sport. Cool-downs should involve jogging and walking alternately until your heart rate is back to normal.

■ Isometric
Isometric exercises such as long-arm bridge pull-overs (»p.128) help to build your core stability and strength, while also offering additional strength gains for the muscles of your arms, shoulders, and upper back.

■ Rotation
Suspended single-arm core rotations (»p.126) increase rotational strength and mobility, providing more force for paddling and rowing. They also stabilize the spine and improve your upper-body strength.

■ Side flexion
Side-lying lateral crunches (»p.80) help to improve your lateral spinal mobility and stability, enabling you to resist external pressures and hold your body in the optimal position for balance and for generating core power.

SWIMMING-BASED SPORTS

Swimming-based sports place significant strain on the muscles, particularly those in the back and shoulders. A flexible spine and good shoulder joints are vital for peak performance.

SPORTS SUCH AS...

- Swimming
- Diving
- Water polo

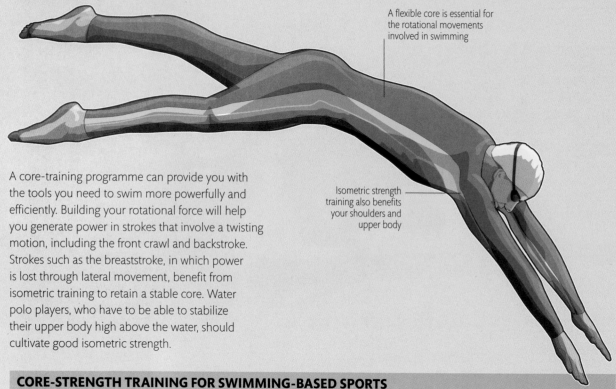

A flexible core is essential for the rotational movements involved in swimming

Isometric strength training also benefits your shoulders and upper body

A core-training programme can provide you with the tools you need to swim more powerfully and efficiently. Building your rotational force will help you generate power in strokes that involve a twisting motion, including the front crawl and backstroke. Strokes such as the breaststroke, in which power is lost through lateral movement, benefit from isometric training to retain a stable core. Water polo players, who have to be able to stabilize their upper body high above the water, should cultivate good isometric strength.

CORE-STRENGTH TRAINING FOR SWIMMING-BASED SPORTS

Endurance and power are essential for swimming. However, the more streamlined your body, the more easily you will move through the water, so strength training for swimming should focus on increasing strength without adding bulk. Using your own bodyweight for resistance, rather than free or machine weights, is best for this.

PREPARATION
Warm-ups for swimming-based sports should include shoulder stretches, ideally with movements that mimic those in swimming, to develop joint mobility. Slow laps and stretches can be used as part of your cool-down.

■ Isometric
Varieties of isometric exercises such as swims (**»p.94**) or planks (**»pp.102–05**) help to build your core stability and strength, enabling you to hold your body in the correct position in the water.

■ Rotation
Rotational exercises such as o-bar rotations (**»pp.114–15**) improve your rotational strength and mobility. These increase the power you can generate in strokes that are based on rotational movements, such as freestyle and backstroke.

■ Extension
Certain extension movements, such as exercise ball back extensions (**»p.122**) improve your spinal mobility and stability. This will help to improve the length of your stroke and the reach of your dives.

CYCLING

Long-distance cycling, sprinting, and stunt cycling, such as BMX biking, all require good balance and an ability to transfer explosive force to the legs from the powerhouse of the core.

Building isometric strength will prepare you for bracing your body against the forces exerted by the varying, uneven terrain you may encounter when cycling. It will also allow you to hold a braced position when going over jumps, increase overall balance, and reduce unwanted sideways movement in your torso when pedalling. Improving your side flexion will help you to lean into corners on the bicycle in situations where you are trying to maximize speed.

A strong core helps you to maintain a good posture when cycling

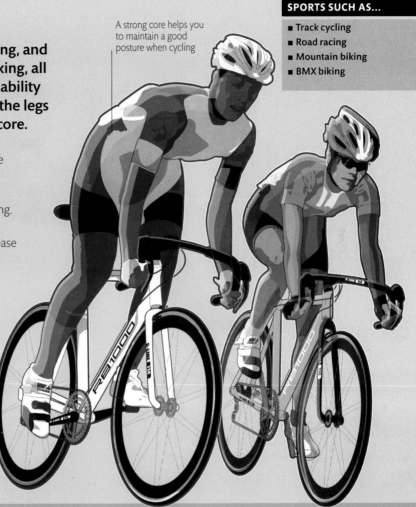

SPORTS SUCH AS...

- Track cycling
- Road racing
- Mountain biking
- BMX biking

CORE-STRENGTH TRAINING FOR CYCLING

Performing strength-training circuits, with an emphasis on leg exercises, develop your explosive power; the more these mimic the types of movement frequently used in cycling, the better. Tightness of the leg muscles is an occupational hazard for cyclists, so make sure you include a comprehensive stretching programme in your training.

PREPARATION
Warm-ups for cycling should involve dynamic stretches that imitate the movements required and to prepare your body for strenuous activity. Cool-downs should involve static stretches to stop your muscles seizing up.

■ **Isometric**
Isometric exercises such as planks (**»pp.102–05**) build core stability, enabling you to hold the correct posture when cycling. These will also help your balance and strength against external forces.

■ **Extension**
Extension exercises like GHD back extensions (**»p.143**) target your spine, lower back, and glutes. These create a core base for driving the pedalling motion, and help re-balance muscles after periods of fixed flexion.

■ **Side flexion**
Side flexion exercises such as heel reaches (**»p.82**) improve your spinal strength and flexibility. This will further improve your posture and pedalling power.

EQUESTRIAN SPORTS

Training for equestrian sports, such as horse racing and showjumping, should concentrate on core strength and spinal agility. Stretching the knees, hips, and back is also vital before spending any time in the saddle.

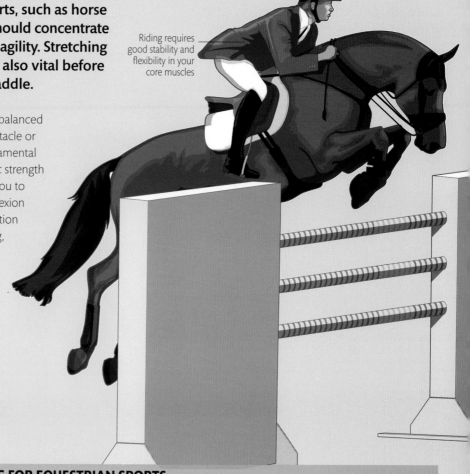

Riding requires good stability and flexibility in your core muscles

Being able to brace your body in a balanced position while jumping over an obstacle or riding across uneven terrain is fundamental to good form. Developing isometric strength to promote core stability will help you to achieve this. Working on your side flexion will allow you to move with the motion of the horse while retaining a strong, stable position in the saddle.

SPORTS SUCH AS...

- **Dressage**
- **Showjumping**
- **Polo**
- **Eventing**
- **Horse racing**
- **Steeplechase**

CORE-STRENGTH TRAINING FOR EQUESTRIAN SPORTS

Training for equestrian activities benefits from the use of strength-training circuits geared towards building your isometric strength. However, other exercise systems with an emphasis on flexibility and core strength, such as yoga or Pilates, can also be incorporated into a training programme for equestrian activities.

PREPARATION

Warm-ups for equestrian sports should involve dynamic stretches that imitate the movements required and to prepare you for strenuous activity. Cool-downs should involve a range of static stretches to reduce muscle tightness.

■ Isometric
Isometric exercises such as supermans (**»pp.70–71**) train your body to stabilize and resist the forces generated by constantly changing direction and hurdling obstacles of varying size.

■ Rotation
Rotation exercises such as hip rolls (**»pp.88–89**) improve spinal mobility and gives you the core strength needed to stay in a stable position in the saddle while constantly changing direction.

■ Side flexion
Side flexion exercises such as side bends (**»p.81**) improve your spinal strength and flexibility. These help your posture and further brace your body against the demands of multidirectional movement.

EXTREME SPORTS

Extreme sports, such as rock climbing, parkour, and skydiving, involve a range of complex, multi-joint movements that exert pressure on a variety of joints and muscles throughout the body.

These activities require excellent mobility and the ability to generate power from a stable position. Improving your side flexion will make it easier for you to reach out to grab awkwardly positioned handholds without compromising your stability. Building your isometric strength will help you to cut out inessential movements, which in turn conserves energy and makes your technique more efficient.

Good flexibility is needed to perform the demanding movements required by extreme sports

SPORTS SUCH AS...

- Rock climbing
- Parkour
- Skydiving
- Ice climbing
- Mountaineering

CORE-STRENGTH TRAINING FOR EXTREME SPORTS

Strength-training circuits for extreme sports should work most of the major muscle groups. Activities such as rock climbing place a heavier demand on your forearms than most other sports, so pay attention to developing their load-bearing capacity. Incorporating a comprehensive stretching routine into your training programme is essential.

PREPARATION
Warm-ups for extreme sports should involve dynamic stretches that imitate the movements required by your particular sport. Cool-downs should involve static stretches to prevent your muscles seizing up.

■ Rotation
Exercises such as suspended single-arm core rotations (**»p.126**) give you the core mobility and strength that you need to repeatedly stretch for handholds, and additional arm and shoulder strength.

■ Isometric
Isometric exercises such as core board rotations (**»p.131**) train your body to brace itself against the changing shape of the environment, whether in the air, on the mountainside, or in the skate park.

■ Flexion
Flexion exercises such as pikes (**»p.139**) help you to develop stamina and strength in your core and hip joints, increasing your ability to walk, run, or climb.

GLOSSARY

Abdominal cylinder A girdle of muscle and *fascia* around the lower torso comprising the *multifidus, transverse abdominis, diaphragm,* and *pelvic floor.*

Abduction A movement that involves pushing a limb away from the body.

Abductor A muscle that functions to push a limb away from the body.

Adduction A movement that involves pulling a limb towards the body.

Adductor A muscle that functions to pull a limb towards the body.

Antagonistic muscles Muscles that are arranged in pairs to carry out *flexion* and *extension* of a joint: one of the pair usually contracts to bend the joint, the other to straighten it.

Anterior The front part or surface, as opposed to the *posterior* (rear).

Barbell A type of *free weight* comprising a bar with weight discs at each end, long enough to be held with a shoulder-width grip. The discs may be fixed, or movable to allow variable weight.

BMI (Body Mass Index) A measure of body fat based on height and weight. It is a useful measure for "average" people but should be used with caution, especially when applied to athletes and other people with considerable muscle bulk.

Box A piece of equipment that can be used to add height to exercises, engaging the core on a more advanced level.

Bridge A common *isometric* core strength exercise, which involves raising the body upwards into a straight line from shoulders to knees, while keeping the feet and shoulders flat on the ground.

Cervical Relating to the neck area.

Cervical spine The first seven vertebrae in the spine, located immediately below the head.

Conditioning A programme of exercise designed to improve performance or prepare for a sporting event.

Cool-down A period of gentle exercise and stretching after a training session, designed to help return the body to its pre-exercise state.

Core The area of the body between the base of the ribs and the hips and buttocks. It stabilizes the *thoracic* cage and pelvis and maintains spinal strength, stability, and mobility. The foundation for all body movement, it provides an axis of power for the *kinetic chain*, and helps to maintain good posture.

Core activation The process of "waking up" the *core*, to ensure that the core muscles are working together properly, and that the correct muscles are being used for each movement.

Core board A piece of equipment used in *stability training* that is used to promote good *core stability* and balance.

Core mobility Movement of the spine and hips.

Core stability Control of the position and movement of the mid-section (trunk).

Crunch A common *flexion* exercise similar to a *sit-up* that involves raising the upper body off the floor towards the lower body.

Deep muscles Muscles that are located beneath the *superficial muscles.*

Diaphragm The muscle that separates the chest cavity from the abdomen.

Diastasis recti A medical condition that can affect pregnant women, during which the muscles of the *rectus abdominis* begin to separate along the central *fascia.*

Drill A practice version of a movement or skill required in sport or activity, usually undertaken as part of training to improve technique.

Dumbbell A type of *free weight* comprising a short bar with a weight disc at each end designed to be lifted with one hand. The weight discs may be fixed or movable to allow variable weight.

Dynamic exercise Any activity in which the joints and muscles are moving.

Erector A muscle that raises a body part.

Erector spinae A group of muscles that run the length of the spine, providing support when you *flex* and *extend.* They are also involved in stabilizing the spine against sideways movement.

Exercise ball A large, inflatable ball that is used in *stability exercises.*

Extensor A muscle that works to increase the angle at a joint – for example straightening the elbow. It usually works in tandem with a *flexor.*

Extension A straightening action. The opposite of *flexion.*

External obliques Surface muscles located on either side of the *rectus abdominis.* They are important to *rotational* core movements and *side flexion.* Together with the *internal obliques,* the muscles also help to stabilize the spine against *lateral* forces.

Facet joint A small joint that connects each vertebra with the vertebra directly above and below it, providing stability to the spine.

Fascia A piece of connective tissue between different muscles.

Fixator muscles See *Neutralizers.*

Flexion Occurs when a muscle is tightened and a limb bends; the opposite of *extension.*

Flexor A muscle that works to decrease the angle at a joint – for example bending the elbow. It usually works in tandem with an *extensor.*

Foam roller A cylindrical piece of equipment made of dense foam used for *mobility exercises* – especially the self-massage of tight muscles.

Free weight A weight – usually a *barbell* or *dumbbell* that is not tethered to a cable or machine.

Frontal plane Also known as the "coronal plane", this divides the body vertically into front and back.

Form The posture or stance used when performing exercises. Good – or correct – form ensures that the exercise is as effective as possible, and helps to prevent injury.

GHD (Glute Hamstring Developer) A piece of exercise equipment designed to work the *gluteals* and hamstrings.

Gluteals The three muscles that make up the buttocks: the *gluteus maximus, gluteus medius,* and *gluteus minimus.*

Gluteus maximus The largest and most *superficial* of the three *gluteal* muscles.

Gluteus medius The second-largest muscle in the buttocks, the gluteus medius lies between the *gluteus maximus,* and the *gluteus minimus,* with which it works to *abduct* the thigh.

Gluteus minimus The smallest of the muscles in the buttocks, the gluteus minimus lies beneath the *gluteus medius,* with which it works to *abduct* the thigh.

Half exercise ball A piece of equipment for instability training exercises that comprises half an exercise ball and a stable platform.

Hip flexors Located within the hip joint, the hip flexors (psoas muscle group) control *flexion* movements in the hips.

Homeostasis The processes by which the body regulates its internal environment to keep conditions stable and constant.

Hypermobile joint A joint that is loosely held together because the ligaments are either naturally lax or have been overstrained.

Hypomobile joint A joint that moves less than it should. This can be caused by shortening of the muscles attached to, or crossing over, the joint.

Interval training A form of training in which short periods of work at near maximal intensity are alternated with periods of rest or lighter exercise, such as brisk walking or jogging.

Isometric A term applied to actions during which the muscles work but do not contract significantly – for example when pushing against an immovable object, or resisting an external force.

Isotonic Training in which muscles work against a constant resistance, so that they contract while the resistance remains the same.

ITB (Iliotibial Band) A tough group of fibres running along the outside of the thigh that primarily works as a stabilizer during running.

Kegel exercises Exercises aimed at improving muscle strength to prevent or remedy problems such as incontinence. Exercises usually involve repeatedly contracting and relaxing the muscles of the *pelvic floor*.

Kettlebell A hand-held metal *free weight* resembling a ball with a handle often used in *plyometric* strength training

Kinetic chain A movement system consisting of myofascial (muscular), articular (joints), and neural (motor) components. Each of these individual components are dependent on the others.

Kyphosis A curvature of the spine that results in bowing or rounding of the back. It often occurs in conjunction with *lordosis*.

Lateral Positioned towards the outside of the body.

Lateral flexion See *side flexion*.

Lateral plane Side-to-side movement.

Lactic acid A waste product of anaerobic respiration. It accumulates in the muscles during intense exercise and is involved in the chemical processes that cause muscular cramp.

Ligament A tough and fibrous connective tissue that connects the bones together at the joints.

Lumbar Relating to the lower back.

Lumbar spine The five vertebrae of the lower back.

Lordosis A common postural problem that occurs when the lumbar curve becomes over-pronounced. Also known as "sway back". It often occurs in conjunction with *kyphosis*.

Medicine ball A weighted ball often used in *plyometric* strength training to build explosive power.

Metabolism The sum of all the body's chemical processes: it comprises anabolism (building up compounds) and catabolism (breaking down compounds).

Mobility exercise An exercise that helps to ease the movement of the joints, or assists a physiotherapist to assess the level of rehabilitation.

Multifidus Muscles in the spine that stabilize the joints.

Neutralizers Also known as synergist or fixator muscles, these help to cancel out any extra movement from other muscles to make sure they move in the correct way.

Neutral hip/pelvis A pelvic position important for good posture that involves it being evenly balanced in relation to the spine and thigh bones.

Neutral spine A position of the spine important for good posture, in which the spine is not completely straight, but has slight curves in the upper and lower regions.

Pelvic floor The area of muscle located in the lower part of the abdomen and attached to the pelvis.

Pike A common *flexion* exercise, which involves bending the body at the hips while keeping the legs and upper body straight.

Plank An *isometric* core strength exercise, which involves holding the body in a straight, immobile position. The most common form is the front plank in which the body is held horizontally with the weight borne on the forearms, elbows, and toes.

Plyometrics Exercises that aim to improve the explosive speed and power of movements by training muscles to contract more quickly and powerfully.

Posterior The back part or surface, as opposed to *anterior*, or front.

Proprioception The term used to describe the information originating in muscles, ligaments, tendons, and joints sent to the brain via the nervous system to provide information about the position and movement of the body.

Quadratus lumborum A core muscle at the base of the trunk involved in *side flexion*.

Rectus abdominis The "six-pack" muscle located at the front of the abdomen, which is involved in *flexion* movements

Rehabilitation The process of recovering from an injury, often with the assistance of sports-medicine professionals such as physiotherapists.

Roman chair A piece of exercise equipment that enables the body to flex at the hips with the feet supported.

Rotation A circular or semi-circular movement around a centre point. Many sports feature significant rotation of body parts including golf, boxing, discus, and hammer.

Sacroiliac joints The two joints located at the base of the back on either side of the spine between the *sacrum* and the ilia (hip bones).

Sacrum A triangular-shaped bone made up of five fused vertebrae, it connects the *lumbar spine* to the coccyx (tailbone).

Sagittal plane A plane that bisects the body down the middle. Moving along the sagittal plane means moving left and right.

Scapula Another term for the shoulder blade.

Scoliosis A medical condition involving the curvature of the spine to one side. It may cause problems with posture, breathing, and walking.

Sensorimotor Relating to processes and activities involving the communication between the brain and the muscles via the nerves.

Set A defined number of repetitions of an exercise used in training.

Side flexion A sideways movement of the spine and/or the core. Also known as *lateral flexion*.

Sit-up A common *flexion* exercise similar to a *crunch* that involves raising the upper body off the floor towards the lower body, usually with both feet flat on the floor and the knees bent.

Slide board A smooth board with adjustable bumpers at either end used in *stability exercises*.

Stabilizers Small muscles close to the spine which hold the vertebrae of the spine in position.

Stability disc A simple inflatable disc that used in *stability exercises*.

Stability exercise An exercise involving an element of instability, such as an unstable surface, to develop the core *stabilizers*.

Static exercise See *Isometric*.

Superficial muscles Muscles located near the surface of the body, which can often be seen through the skin in people with low body fat.

Suspension band A piece of stability exercise *training* equipment that is suspended from a rack or other stable piece of gym equipment, and suspends one or more limbs in the air to make the exercise more challenging.

Thoracic Relating to the area of the chest and back positioned between the neck and lumbar regions.

Thoracic spine The longest portion of the spinal column, made up of the middle 12 vertebrae.

Tendon A type of connective tissue that joins the muscles to the bones, and transmits the force of muscle contraction to the bones.

Transverse abdominis A deep muscle that runs around the abdomen, acting like a girdle to hold the muscles of the core together.

Transverse plane A plane bisecting the body horizontally through the abdomen.

Warm-up A series of low-intensity exercises used to prepare the body for a workout by moderately stimulating the heart, lungs, and muscles. These normally involve a combination of dynamic exercises and low-intensity cardiovascular work.

INDEX

ACKNOWLEDGMENTS

About the authors

Glen Thurgood MSc is Head of Athletic Performance at The Rugby Football Club and the owner of GTSportsPerformance (www.gtsportsperformance.com). With over 12 years' combined experience as an elite athlete and coach, he has worked with rugby union, football, and baseball teams at university, professional, and national levels.

Mary Paternoster is an established Pilates teacher and has trained with some of the world's leading professionals. She is the owner of Infinite Conditioning (www.infiniteconditioning.com) a Pilates personal training company based in London. With over 12 years' professional dance, personal training and Pilates coaching experience, she also runs educational workshops for independent wellness companies and advises corporate coaching companies in the UK and Europe.

Author and publisher acknowledgments

The authors and publishers would like to thank the following people and organizations for their generous help in producing this book.

For modelling:
Mary Paternoster; Glen Thurgood; Ben Gollings; Lauren Gollings; Gareth Saptead; Gareth Jones; Scott Tindall; Chris Chea; Michelle Grey; Anouska Hipperson; Megan Lols; Juan King; Albert Raper; Rufus Shosman.

For use of facilities:
Tom Haynes, Becky Littlewood and Sian Bates at The Training Shed (www.trainingshed.com), Daventry for use of their fantastic facilities and patience during the photoshoot; Phil Littlewood at indigo23 (www.indigo23.co.uk) for use of their superb training equipment.

For reference photography:
Cobalt ID; Phil Gamble.

For illustrations:
Philip Wilson; Debbie Maizels; Phil Gamble; Mark Walker; Debajyoti Dutta; Mike Garland; Darren R. Awuah; Jon Rogers.

For additional material and assistance:
Phil Gamble (additional work on illustrations); Margaret McCormack (Indexing); Priyanka Singh, Vidit Vashisht (Design); Suparna Sengupta, Pallavi Singh (Editorial).

SAFETY INFORMATION

All physical activity involves a potential risk of injury. Participants must therefore take all reasonable care during exercise. Any training programme should be carried out under the guidance of the appropriate professionals, and participants should also seek the advice of their doctor, or equivalent healthcare professional, before beginning any form of exercise.

The publishers of this book and its contributors are confident that the exercises described herein, when performed correctly, with gradual increases in resistance and proper supervision, are safe. However, readers of this book must ensure that the equipment and facilities they use for their training are fit for purpose, and they should adhere to safety guidelines at times, including both those outlined in this book and any required by the manufactures and/or owners of the facilities. They should also ensure that supervisors have adequate insurance and relevant, up-to-date accreditations and qualifications, including emergency first aid.

The publishers, consultant editors, and contributing authors of this book take no responsibility for injury to persons or property consequent on embarking upon the advice and guidelines included herein.